On the Rocks

On the Rocks

Straight Talk about Women and Drinking

Susan D. Stewart

ROWMAN & LITTLEFIELD
Lanham • Boulder • New York • London

Published by Rowman & Littlefield
An imprint of The Rowman & Littlefield Publishing Group, Inc.
4501 Forbes Boulevard, Suite 200, Lanham, Maryland 20706
www.rowman.com

86-90 Paul Street, London EC2A 4NE

British Library Cataloguing in Publication Information Available

Library of Congress Cataloging-in-Publication Data On File

ISBN: 978-1-5381-2725-4 (cloth)
ISBN: 978-1-5381-2726-1 (electronic)

Contents

Acknowledgments

I am indebted to the women who shared their thoughts, stories, and some-times painful aspects of their lives, without whom this work would not have been possible.

Note on the COVID-19 Pandemic

All interviews were conducted in the summer of 2019, roughly nine months prior to widespread lockdowns associated with COVID-19. The pandemic has altered the way we live in fundamental ways: the way we work, interact with others, perform our daily routines, and engage in behaviors related to our health and well-being. A number of studies found a surge in alcohol sales since the outbreak.[1] For example, a survey by Nielsen found that alcohol sales were more than 50 percent higher in March of 2020 than in March of 2019.[2] Studies based on nationally representative samples of Americans showed significant increases in alcohol consumption (with Australia, Norway, Belgium, Spain, and other Western countries experiencing similar increases).[3] While suffering associated with COVID-19 has been widespread, the pandemic has taken an especially heavy toll on women. They are disproportionately employed in service occupations that experienced massive layoffs, and were more likely to leave their jobs to be at home with their children. Whether employed or not, women found themselves primarily or solely responsible for their children's remote learning, the care of relatives, housework, and overall household management. This was the case even among married women and those with a male partner in the home. There is growing alarm as to how COVID-19 is affecting women with children, who are widely viewed as being under particularly stressful conditions since the pandemic. Jokes and memes about mothers' increased reliance on alcohol to cope have exploded on social media since the pandemic. In June of 2020, in the midst of writing this book, I conducted an online survey of 546 women about their use of alcohol since the pandemic, as well as their psychological well-being (e.g., life satisfaction, depression, anxiety, and stress), and, for those with children, their parenting experiences (e.g., parenting stress, parent-child closeness). My findings were consistent with those of other studies. Nearly two-thirds of respondents reported drinking more since the beginning of the pandemic, including increases in daily drinking, drinking earlier in the day, and binge drinking. Results were similar among women with children. Coronavirus-related anxiety and parenting stress were associated with increased drinking.[4] Other studies have found strong linkages between pandemic-related stressors and alcohol consumption among both women and men.[5] Researchers are continuing to track alcohol use during the pandemic, with the hope that the increase will subside with widespread vaccinations, the opening back up of businesses and schools, reunions between family members, and reduction in sickness and death. However, the long-term effects of the pandemic on many facets of life are unknown, and a return to what we thought of as "normalcy" is unlikely.

Chapter One

Stormy Seas

TRACY: I can't think of a single engagement in my adult life that has not been surrounded by or included alcohol ever. I can't think of a single one. Oh my gosh.

—Tracy, age 36, project manager

American women are swimming in a sea of alcohol, and we are letting them drown. Rows of flavored vodkas line the shelves of grocery stores: lime, tangerine, cinnamon, and even coffee, as do wines called Middle Sister, Cupcake, Little Black Dress, and Mad Housewife, just to name a few. On social media, jokes and memes about how much women drink abound. Wine glasses that hold a whole bottle of wine so women can say they only had "one glass." Purses and baby bags that dispense wine. Alcohol-themed T-shirts, greeting cards, magnets, mugs, dish towels, you name it. There is even wine ice cream. More sinister yet, wine is being marketed with "pink ribbons" ostensibly to fight breast cancer, when studies consistently show that even moderate alcohol use increases breast cancer risk. These days, excessive drinking among women is seen as a source of amusement. Amy Schumer guzzling boxed wine in hit movies such as *Trainwreck*. Alcohol-themed movies such as *Girls' Night Out*, *Rough Night*, and *Girls Trip* were all released within a single year. More recently, TikTok has become a popular platform for stressed-out moms to post jokey videos about their drinking. And one cannot talk about the influence of the media on women's use of alcohol without mentioning the HBO show *Sex and the City*, which featured four single, educated, career women downing "cosmos" while commiserating over work, love, and life at the dawn of a new millennium. Increasingly, alcohol has become central to women's identities and expressions of self, and is seen as a necessary part of leisure activities. "Book club night" has become a euphemism for "women getting together to drink wine." Book optional.

Women's current level of alcohol consumption is no laughing matter. Americans, both men and women, are drinking at unprecedented levels. According to Gallup, nearly two-thirds (65 percent) of Americans said they drink alcoholic beverages, 29 percent of whom reported having had a drink in the last twenty-four hours. Among drinkers, 13 percent said they drank eight or more drinks in the last seven days. And although the percentage of adults who say they drink has remained relatively constant, men and women are consuming alcohol more frequently and are drinking more drinks per week. The weekly average number of drinks consumed in 2021 was 3.6, compared to 2.8 in 1996, a 43 percent increase.[1]

According to Herbert Fingarette in his book *Heavy Drinking: The Myth of Alcoholism as a Disease*, in the Colonial era it was common for men and women to consume alcohol, and that Americans drank "far more" alcohol then than we do now.[2] Alcohol was thought to have numerous health benefits for the body and mind and was used to treat all manner of ailments. Moreover, women and men drank alcohol at similar rates and most started drinking as children. Back then, the overuse of alcohol was considered simply "too much of a good thing," as opposed to a disease. With the advent of industrialization and modern science in the nineteenth century, public attitudes toward alcohol shifted. Alcohol was increasingly blamed for numerous societal ills such as poverty and crime, and the use of alcohol dropped by roughly half. The temperance movement, which argued against alcohol consumption of any kind, took hold and led to the Eighteenth Amendment to the Constitution in 1919, the nationwide constitutional ban on the production, importation, and sales of alcoholic beverages, lasting until 1933 (i.e., "Prohibition"). This effort was driven in part by first-wave feminists with the goal of reducing domestic violence and husbands "drinking away" their paychecks.

Paradoxically, the 1920s were also a period of increased drinking among women. Paid employment and the invention of the automobile allowed women more freedom to explore the world away from the watchful eye of parents. Despite continued societal fretting over dangers of alcohol, including the introduction of the term "alcoholism" and the founding of Alcoholics Anonymous (A.A.), the use of alcohol increased steadily among both women and men over the twentieth century.[3] Women experienced especially dramatic growth that has continued into the twenty-first. The increase coincided with women's continued movement into the labor force, increasing education, the sexual revolution, and a similar upward trend in women's alcohol consumption occurred in other Western countries.[4] Alcohol's place in American society became firmly reestablished.

WOMEN'S GROWING USE OF ALCOHOL

Although women drink less alcohol than do men,[5] women's and men's alcohol use has largely converged in terms of prevalence, amount, and frequency, and alcohol-related problems and harms.[6] According to the National Epidemiological Survey on Alcohol and Related Conditions, women experienced a 16 percent increase in past-year alcohol use, a 58 percent increase in high-risk drinking, and an 84 percent increase in alcohol use disorder between 2002 and 2013.[7] A meta-analysis of six U.S. surveys indicated a 23 percent increase in binge drinking among women between 2000 and 2016, with no corresponding increase for men.[8] Male and female high school students' likelihood of binge drinking has also converged in recent years.[9] And it is important to note that alcohol use is notoriously underreported, by as much as 50 percent, with women more likely to underreport drinking behavior than are men.[10]

My key reason for writing this book is to answer this question: *What about women's lives has changed such that they drink more alcohol?* Given the significant increase in women's alcohol consumption, there has been surprisingly little research on this question and explanations for the rise have been for the most part anecdotal. Societal-level reasons put forth by commentators include loss of hope at the state of our economy, low expectations for social mobility, erosion of the safety net, isolation of rural and inner-city communities, depression about the political state of our country, and the fact that alcohol, unlike other mind- and body-altering substances, is easy to access and has far fewer legal restrictions.[11] Others have put in that the use of alcohol has become normalized, permeating just about every aspect of our lives: at home, work, and previously alcohol-free social activities.[12] Independent and art-house movie theaters market themselves as genteel and cultured by offering alcohol—and larger chains such as Cinemark have recently followed suit. Half-marathons and 5Ks now routinely provide beer tents at the finish line. On the *Today* show, Hoda Kotb and Kathy Lee Gifford drank wine at 10 a.m. (While I was writing this book, Jenna Bush Hager replaced Kathy Lee on the show. After she was chastised by her mother, former first lady Laura Bush, the wine glasses were quietly replaced by coffee mugs. Jenna's father, former president George W. Bush, used to be a heavy drinker and maintains he has not had a drink in decades).[13]

Specific to women, in a study by the Caron Treatment Center, women listed stress and anxiety, trouble with romantic relationships, pressure from family and friends, traumatic experiences, and boredom as the top five reasons why they drink.[14] Numerous other studies indicate that women use alcohol to cope with stress.[15] There has also been increasing awareness of the toll persistent microaggressions (i.e., subtle displays of sexism) take on women.

For example, women who perceive they are victims of discrimination are more likely to have an alcohol use disorder.[16] As women continue to break barriers in education and employment, they may use alcohol to be perceived as sophisticated and as powerful.[17] Women are moving into professions where alcohol use is common, in business, law, and tech. Drinking is viewed as an opportunity to bond with colleagues and is often encouraged and facilitated by employers.[18] The former U.S. assistant surgeon general, Rear Admiral Susan Blumenthal, says that much like smoking fifty years ago, alcohol "has become a women's rights tragedy."[19] In the 1960s, Nora Ephron (writer of *When Harry Met Sally* and *Sleepless in Seattle*) was a young reporter at the *New York Post*, one of only several female reporters at the newspaper. She said in her memoir, *I Remember Nothing*, "I was in love with journalism. I loved the city room. I loved the pack. I loved smoking and drinking scotch and playing dollar poker." She says of the 1950s and 1960s, "They didn't drink wine then," and "Wine didn't use to be 'a thing.'"[20]

Although women who drink still experience significantly greater societal disapproval than do men, the stigma attached to women's use of alcohol has diminished.[21] Largely gone are negative portrayals of women drinkers as homeless bag ladies, "loose women," and, conversely "masculine" women (although alcohol use among women with children remains heavily scrutinized, as does alcohol use during pregnancy).[22] The stigma associated with women's drinking may even be reversing, with women increasingly feeling the need to justify why they *don't* drink.[23] Conversations with women who drink suggest they do so to be perceived as more interesting, accomplished, and cool.[24] Television and movies equate drinking with women "cutting loose" and having fun times, harkening back to women's adolescence and college days before the stresses of work, husbands, and children. Women still need to be careful, however. Whereas wine and seltzer-type drinks are considered classy and feminine, women who drink beer or hard liquor are viewed less positively. As is often the case, women must walk a fine line between "good girl" and "wild woman."

There has also been an increase in aggressive marketing of alcohol to women, especially wine, and this is having an effect.[25] Numerous studies indicate that alcohol advertising increases consumption.[26] Americans most commonly consume beer (38 percent), followed by wine (30 percent), and liquor (29 percent).[27] Over half (52 percent) of women say their preferred drink is wine compared to 20 percent of men. The preference for wine among women increased 9 percentage points between 1994 and 2013.[28] According to data gathered by *Beverage Dynamics* magazine, wine's segment of the alcohol market is growing relative to beer and liquor, with younger women driving the increase. Millennials are the largest and fastest-growing group of wine drinkers, easily surpassing both Generation X and baby boomers. Over a third (36 percent) of all wine is consumed by millennials, and the percentage of millennial wine drinkers increased 10 percent in two years. They also consume more wine than other generations, with an average of three glasses per occasion compared to two for Gen-Xers and baby boomers. Whereas "occasional" wine drinking is down, "high frequency" wine drinking (those who have wine daily or multiple times per week) is up.[29] However, the alcohol market is shifting. Blatantly sexist alcohol advertising is declining, and the sales of spiked seltzers such as White Claw and Truly have increased dramatically, driven by millennials and Gen X, and what marketers refer to as a "post-gender world."[30]

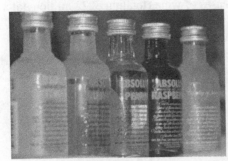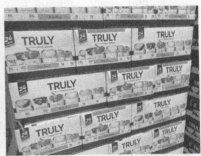

Are brands capitalizing on women's increased use of alcohol, or are they creating a new market of consumers? *Source left*: Ben Sutherland, https://www.flickr.com/photos /60179301@N00/5291229689. *Source right*: Joni Hanebutt/Alamy Stock Photo, Image ID: 2BPBPNC

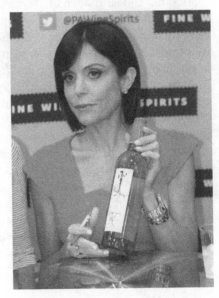

Bethany Frankle, inventor of Skinny Girl adult beverages. *Source*: WENN Rights Ltd/Alamy Stock Photo, Image ID: HDD31K

Alcohol is also more widely available than in the past. There are state-level restrictions on when and where alcohol can be sold, but most have been repealed over the decades (aside from age). For example, the majority of states now allow alcohol to be sold on Sunday.[31] Alcohol is increasingly being purchased for home use as opposed to being consumed at restaurants and bars. The switch to home use of alcohol in recent years is a result of the poor economy and the increase in "fast casual" dining that does not serve alcohol. Older women, less comfortable with the "bar scene," are more likely to drink at home.[32] Direct-to-consumer sales (i.e., wine clubs) rose 8.1 percent between 2014 and 2015, with these online businesses currently making around $2 billion in sales.[33] COVID-19 has only increased at-home alcohol consumption with one million more cases of wine (totaling $222 million dollars) shipped in the first half of 2020 compared to 2019.[34] Alcohol industry trade groups responsible for regulating alcohol marketing have been lax in enforcing rules that companies not promote excessive drinking, especially regarding ads on social media and product placement in movies.[35] Drinking is a common subject of social-media lifestyle "influencers."[36]

ISN'T A GLASS OF WINE GOOD FOR YOU?

No. Drinking is not good for you, even in moderation. Although a number of studies (most conducted decades ago and based on men) point to the health benefits of moderate alcohol consumption, a study of 195 countries and territories, the Global Burden of Disease, suggests that no amount of alcohol is healthy.[37] The negative effects of alcohol use and abuse cannot be understated. Harmful alcohol consumption is the fifth leading cause of death and disability worldwide,[38] and alcohol is expected to continue to be a leading cause of death among men and women in the United States.[39] According to the National Institute of Alcohol Abuse and Alcoholism (NIAAA), alcohol-related deaths currently kill roughly 95,000 American adults (approximately 68,000 men and 27,000 women) per year, making alcohol the third-leading preventable cause of death in the United States. Alcohol-impaired driving accounts for 28 percent of overall driving fatalities.[40] The negative effects of alcohol on physical and mental health include obesity, cancer, dementia, depression, and suicide, and deaths from cirrhosis and alcohol-related liver disease increased 65 percent between 1999 and 2016.[41] More than one in ten (14 percent) of all adults report alcohol use consistent with an alcohol use disorder (AUD) based on meeting at least two of the eleven *Diagnostic and Statistical Manual of Mental Disorders-5* (DSM-5) alcohol abuse criteria.[42] Alcohol-related emergency room visits increased 47 percent between 2006 and 2014.[43]

The U.S. Department of Health and Human Services estimates there are 5.3 million women in the U.S. who are heavy drinkers or who "drink in a way that threatens their health, safety, and general well-being."[44] Alcohol-related cirrhosis increased 50 percent in women between 2009 and 2015. They are also being diagnosed at younger ages than in the past, at a mean age of fifty-four.[45] Nearly a quarter of women (23 percent) reported previous lifetime levels of alcohol use consistent with an alcohol use disorder, and 10 percent within the past twelve months.[46] Women are more susceptible to alcohol-related health conditions and deaths than are men; they have smaller bodies, experience hormonal fluctuations, and have different stomach enzymes with which to process alcohol. These risks persist even adjusting for weight. Alcohol use is linked to alcohol dependence, psychiatric disorders, infertility and reproductive problems, and breast cancer.[47] There has been a greater increase in deaths due to alcoholic liver disease among women than men.[48] An analysis of U.S. death certificates filed between 1999 and 2017 showed an 85 percent increase in deaths due to alcohol among women compared to an increase of only 35 percent for men; among adults twenty-five to sixty-four, the increase was more than three times higher.[49] So-called "deaths of despair," deaths due to alcohol, suicide, and drug overdoses, are responsible for increased death rates and the notable 2015 reversion in U.S. life expectancy for both men and women.[50]

Given these scary but unfortunately true statistics, alcohol use among women warrants a great deal more attention than it has been getting. One estimate suggests that only 8 percent of substance use research has focused specifically on women.[51] Doctors and therapists generally lack specific training in identifying alcohol problems and don't have up-to-date information on treatment options. For example, few American doctors prescribe drugs designed to curb alcohol cravings, such as naltrexone, which is used widely in Europe.[52] Although intake forms are increasingly asking about alcohol and drug use, many doctors are uncomfortable with talking about alcohol and may not know what to do aside from recommending A.A. The concept of "alcoholism as a disease" and the focus on individual failings promoted by A.A. ignore important contextual factors unique to women's lives, such as discrimination in the workplace, motherhood, and shame. As Gabrielle Glaser explains in *Her Best Kept Secret*, A.A., created by upper-middle-class white men in the 1930s, remains largely a male space. She argues that women who attend A.A. meetings are vulnerable to exploitation by men. For instance, immediately finding and having a close relationship with a previously unknown "sponsor" is an important part of the program.[53] Moreover, A.A. is not a science-based treatment; few rigorous studies have been conducted and samples are notoriously biased toward "success." The results of even well-designed studies have been mixed, especially when it comes to women.[54] Yet, in the absence of alternatives, women are forced to take part in "mainstream" treatments (i.e., twelve-step programs and A.A.).[55] Overall, alcohol use disorders remain poorly understood and stigmatized with only vague references to "rehab," "treatment," and "recovery." Only one in five people with an alcohol use disorder has ever been treated, with rates even lower for women.[56]

Overall, Americans are deeply ambivalent about alcohol. In 2020, 86 percent of Americans saw drinking alcohol as morally acceptable as opposed to morally wrong, up from 78 percent in 2018, and 71 percent felt that drinking alcohol in moderation (one or two drinks a day) is either good for your health (16 percent) or makes no difference (55 percent). Yet, 86 percent of Americans viewed alcohol as a problem to society, ranging from a "somewhat serious" problem (39 percent), to a "very serious" problem (29 percent), to an "extremely serious" problem (18 percent), and 79 percent think it is important for government programs to address health risks.[57] More than seven million children, one in ten, live with a parent who has an AUD, around a million of whom live with a single mother.[58] Alcohol is associated with child abuse, neglect, poor child mental health, behavior disorders, adverse childhood experiences, interpersonal violence, low marital quality, higher marital disagreement, and higher marital instability.[59] Over a third (36 percent) of Americans said drinking has been a cause of "trouble in your family."[60] Moreover, few recognize the negative economic impact of alcohol use such as higher unemployment, reduced work productivity, more absences, and workplace accidents and injuries.[61]

SOCIOECONOMIC DIVERSITY IN WOMEN'S ALCOHOL USE

The common stereotype of "women who drink" is that they are poor, uneducated, and non-white. The reality is that lower-income women are less likely to consume alcohol than are higher-income women. The same goes for women of color and women with lower levels of education.[62] This includes binge drinking.[63] In a study of white women, one-third of those with a four-year college degree drank multiple times per week (31 percent), compared to 21 percent with some college and 14 percent with a high school diploma.[64] This same pattern has been observed among European women.[65]

The reasons are not completely clear, but some speculate that higher income groups, in addition to having more discretionary income to purchase alcohol, have greater opportunities to participate in activities that involve alcohol, such as dining out and vacations. Likely related to income, suburban dwellers drink more than those in cities, and more than those in small towns and rural areas. A slightly higher percentage of liberals and Democrats drink than conservatives, moderates, Republicans, and independents. People who are employed and people who attend church least drink more frequently and in greater amounts than those who are not employed and/or are regular churchgoers.[66]

Alcohol consumption also varies greatly by women's race and ethnicity. The Centers for Disease Control (CDC) measures alcohol use and related problems in various ways, and no matter what the measure, white women have the highest levels of drinking and alcohol-related harms than other racial and ethnic groups, aside from American Indians and Alaskan Natives.[67] There are differences among non-white, non-Hispanic women, with Black and Hispanic women drinking somewhat more than Asians. Data from the National Health Interview Survey showed that 47 percent of Black, 41 percent of Hispanic, and 37 percent of Asian women said they drank at least monthly, compared to 71 percent of whites. Eleven percent of Hispanic, 17 percent of Black, and 19 percent of Asian women drank multiple days per week, versus 27 percent of white women. Twenty-seven percent of Hispanic, 23 percent of Black, and 16 percent of Asian women reported alcohol consumption consistent with binge drinking compared to 33 percent of white women.[68]

There has been a particularly large increase in deaths due to alcohol among white women specifically. Death certificate data showed that between 1999 and 2016, non-Hispanic white women age twenty-five to sixty-four experienced a 120 percent increase in alcohol-induced causes of deaths, followed by American Indians/Alaskan Natives at 72 percent and Hispanics at 39 percent. African American women experienced a decline of 19 percent.[69] Similarly, data from the National Emergency Department Sample (NEDS) indicates that deaths due to alcohol have increased 130 percent among white women since 1999. This compares to an increase of 27 percent for Hispanic women and a decrease of 27 percent for Black women.[70] Lower levels of education and income among women of color may underlie these differences—an analysis of data from the National Longitudinal Survey of Youth 1979 (NLSY79), conducted by myself with colleagues, showed similar levels of drinking among college graduates regardless of race and ethnicity.[71] In other research, Hispanic women who have adopted the attitudes of mainstream culture had higher levels of alcohol consumption than less-assimilated women.[72]

DRINKING ACROSS THE LIFECOURSE

A developmental perspective of alcohol use stresses that "variability in drinking patterns is not constant across the lifespan, and that pressures to drink—or not to drink—are concentrated at certain stages in the course of a person's life."[73] Indeed, a woman's use of alcohol over her lifetime, or her *drinking trajectory*, is particularly sensitive to lifecourse transitions. According to researchers Nicole Laborde and Christina Mair, women "mature out of drinking behaviors once they enter traditional adult roles . . . perhaps due to social expectations and/or additional responsibilities that make heavy drinking difficult."[74] Whereas some transitions have been shown to be protective against alcohol use—gaining steady employment, marriage, impending pregnancy and parenthood—others, such as attending college, divorce, and children leaving the nest are associated with higher rates.[75] Overall, alcohol consumption declines with age.[76] Yet, the pressure not to drink among older women appears to be diminishing, and alcohol consumption and hazardous drinking have increased dramatically among women at midlife and beyond.[77] Three decades ago, the alcohol research team Sharon and Richard Wilsnack foretold that women would become increasingly likely to develop chronic drinking problems because their lives are decreasingly likely to be interrupted by life changes associated with less drinking.[78]

In the end, there is a lot we don't know about why women are drinking more. Due to many factors—stigma, shame, denial, fear of having children taken away and losing one's job—women who have problems with alcohol, or who have the potential to have problems, remain largely hidden from view. Current approaches to substance abuse, including alcohol, are not particularly helpful in this regard. For example, women with children generally don't have the luxury of going away for a month of treatment (let alone paying for it—inpatient treatment is rarely fully covered by insurance), so expanding the availability of inpatient programs would likely be ineffective. In a study of one hundred mothers who completed treatment for addiction, reasons they gave for not seeking treatment earlier included: I was afraid to leave my family, I was concerned about the social stigma and its impact on my family, I thought I could control it myself, I didn't think I had a problem, and I felt I had no one to take care of my children if I went into treatment.[79] Then too, many women are economically dependent upon husbands and partners who have drinking problems themselves.[80]

Are we not noticing women's growing use of alcohol, or are we *choosing* not to notice? Arguably, women, and especially mothers, hold together the whole fabric of society at home, at work, and in their communities. Any threat to mothers is a threat to us all, and the thought that something might be "wrong" with mothers may lead us to look the other way. Women's use of alcohol and other substances is not new. Betty Friedan's *The Feminine Mystique* was the first to highlight the emptiness and depression felt by middle-class, suburban housewives of the 1950s and 1960s who were thought to "have it all."[81] In those days, depressed women were quietly prescribed "mother's little helper," mainly Valium and other sedatives. As far back as the 1800s, doctors gave morphine to women to relieve symptoms from a range of ailments including menstrual cramps, morning sickness, and "diseases of a nervous character." This led some women down the path of addiction. However, before the widespread criminalization of drugs and restrictions on alcohol, substance use among women was considered a "scandal" as opposed to a crime.[82]

There has been increasing public awareness of women's, especially mothers', increased use of alcohol. Most of the attention is coming from mothers themselves. Scary Mommy, a popular motherhood website that's part informational and part confessional, has published numerous stories on this: "Scary mommy confessions: When you're a mom who drinks," "This is why a mom needs wine," "Other moms tell me to drink, and this is why it matters," and "How I handle motherhood without alcohol." There are literally hundreds of memoirs about women and alcohol use disorders: *Blackout*, *Lit*, *Drinking: A Love Story*, and *Smashed* to name a few. *Mommy Doesn't Drink Here Anymore* and *Diary of an Alcoholic Housewife* chronicle two mothers' experiences quitting drinking. Movies have tended to stay away from this topic, choosing to celebrate alcohol use as opposed to condemning it. However, there are several that attempt to realistically portray women with alcohol use disorders, such as *28 Days* with Sandra Bullock and *When a Man Loves a Woman* with Meg Ryan. There is no lack of books that trivialize alcohol use. One of the most famous is *Sippy Cups Are Not for Chardonnay*, a funny, mom-to-mom look at the ups and downs of raising children (the author later admitted to having a "problem" with alcohol).[83] *Mommy's Favorite Juice*, a book for children, is described as "an endearing tale of a young son, Max, who inspires his mother to dream of an evening of peace and quiet and her favorite juice (wine). Follow Max and his mother as they travel to the store and learn about the different colors of Mommy's juice and why Mommy is not allowed any juice before dinner. Thirsty mothers everywhere will enjoy reading this book with their children every day." (I'm sorry, but *WTF?*).

THEORETICAL PERSPECTIVES

Aside from an underlying feminist perspective, this book is guided by a developmental perspective, namely lifecourse theory. The lifecourse focuses on how people's choices are embedded in a set of opportunities and constraints such as their economic status, family background, political systems, and historical times. Although events outside one's control can disrupt a person's anticipated trajectory through life, individuals do have agency, with ability to "construct their own lifecourse." Peoples' lives *unfold*, with development not stopping at the end of childhood but continuing through the end of life. For example, husbands' and wives' alcohol use is highly correlated and alcohol is a key component of assortative mating, although women's drinking is more heavily influenced by their partner's drinking than vice versa.[84] Current choices and actions affect subsequent ones, and transitions in one person's life affect the people around them.[85] They also affect those of people not even born, and norms, values, and behaviors are transmitted across generations.[86] Attitudes and behaviors about alcohol and drinking are taught (and learned) through the family, peers, the media, school curricula, churches, and the legal system. For example, a family history of alcohol-related problems (beyond genetics) is associated with higher levels of alcohol use and alcohol use disorders.[87]

Similarly, ecological theory views individuals as embedded in a system of relationships in which one person's attitudes, experiences, and behavior reverberate across a shared social network.[88] Women are the main caretakers of not only children but aging parents and extended family members, a group known as the Sandwich Generation.[89] There is a distinct lack of information on women's use of alcohol beyond adolescence and young adulthood. Midlife women in particular are at the top of their professions and productivity as workers and earners. They are the first to step up to meet the needs of their communities; their unpaid labor makes substantial contributions to the greater good *free of charge*.[90] Behaviors that threaten women's physical and socioemotional health, such as drinking (on their part or on the part of others in their lives), will no doubt have lasting effects across the family system, between generations, and on society as a whole.

A final theory drawn upon in this book is that of family stress. Family stress is a physical and psychological response to "stressors," defined as life events, occurrences, and transitions of sufficient magnitude as to bring about change in the family system.[91] Stressors can be acute (e.g., retirement, job loss), chronic (e.g., marital problems, ailing parents), or simply "everyday hassles" (e.g., losing car keys, forgetting something at the store). Either way, family stress theory is concerned with understanding individuals' adaptation and adjustment to stressors and the role of various resources (e.g., family support) and liabilities (e.g., low income).[92] Stressors large and small have been linked to poorer child, adult, and family outcomes and use of substances, including alcohol. For example, a study of Australian women found drinking intentions and behavior were related to "having a stressful week" and because it "makes me feel relaxed."[93]

Women's roles have expanded, multiplied, and become more demanding, as the result of rising expectations for children (and mothers), and increases in women's education, employment, and income.[94] Most American women are juggling paid work and family caregiving. Stress related to employment is associated with increased alcohol use.[95] Conflict between work and family demands is associated with worse physical and psychological health and greater use of alcohol among women.[96]

WHY I WROTE THIS BOOK

I found these trends troubling and developed a heightened awareness of the way that alcohol was being portrayed on television, movies, and social media, and how alcohol was being consumed within my own social circle. It turns out that women who drink, and who may be teetering on the edge of harmful drinking, look the same as other women. They get up, go to work, make dinner, do laundry, make doctor's appointments, plan parties, and otherwise carry out a never-ending list of activities needed to maintain hearth and home (and look good while doing it). They do these things every day without fail. I wanted to delve deeper into the role of alcohol in women's lives than newspaper stories, Facebook posts, and statistical studies allow. This is not, and was never intended to be, a study of women with alcohol use disorders or women in recovery. By all rights the women in my study could be considered "regular gals," and the amount of alcohol they said they consume, and the way they consume it, is consistent with national data. Nor is this book a condemnation of women who enjoy drinking, drink to celebrate, or even drink to cope. Quite the opposite. Despite the dire warnings, I provide no judgment regarding the "right" amount of alcohol women should be consuming, or when, or how. (There is no consensus among scientists anyway.) My purpose is to provide a look at women's perceptions of alcohol in their lives and in society at large. Serendipitously, my study happened to occur at a point in time exactly one century from the largest sustained discussion of alcohol American society has ever had (i.e., Prohibition). What's different is that *women* are the primary subject of the conversation.

RESEARCH METHODOLOGY

The participants in the study are women age twenty-five and older who drink alcohol at least occasionally. The women were recruited from a midwestern metropolitan area with a total population of roughly 650,000. Women under the age of twenty-five were excluded because of the temporary upswing in drinking and binge drinking among this group. Participants were primarily recruited through flyers posted in places where women tend to congregate (daycares, health clubs, libraries, etc.) and through social media, such as through "moms" Facebook groups. Other participants were recruited through snowball sampling using networks of women connected to one another through their children's various academic, social, and sports activities. Given the remaining stigma around women and alcohol, I used a "normative approach" to attract a wide range of women. That is, flyers, announcements, and other recruitment materials were designed to normalize (and not stigmatize) women's drinking. I included images of women and alcohol typically found in the media that portray drinking in a neutral or somewhat positive light. These strategies yielded thirty-two participants, at which point saturation was achieved.

Individual face-to-face interviews were conducted over the summer of 2019. Before the interview, participants completed a Qualtrics survey on their phones, where they recorded their sociodemographic characteristics and patterns of alcohol use. There were two sets of questions pertaining to alcohol consumption. The first module contained a standard set of alcohol consumption questions developed by the NIAAA Task Force on Recommended Alcohol Questions.[97] The second module assessed alcohol abuse based on the DSM-5, which is the standard mechanism for diagnosing alcohol use disorders.[98] The survey gathered basic demographic information from participants including their age, race/ethnicity, education, employment, occupation, income, relationship status, religious affiliation and spirituality, religious service attendance, and children (number, age, gender, relationship, and residence). The survey allowed space for written comments.

Grounded theory methodology formed the basis of the qualitative analysis, in which ideas, terms, concepts, and themes are allowed to emerge naturally from the data. I have integrated my findings with theoretical, qualitative, and quantitative research pulled from the gender, family, medical, public health, and policy literature. With the assistance of NVivo software, transcriptions were coded to identify and bring together relevant passages, concepts, ideas, and other groupings. Throughout my analysis, I practiced "reflexivity," in that my own subjective commitments, experiences, and feelings were "acknowledged, confronted, and integrated" into the analysis. Quotes were edited for clarity when I felt it was necessary; for example, I generally removed "ums," "likes," and abrupt stops and starts. Participants' names were replaced with pseudonyms, and information that could potentially identify participants and their families was removed or altered.

CHARACTERISTICS OF PARTICIPANTS

My intention was never to attempt to interview a representative sample of women, especially given the racial and ethnic homogeneity of the region. However, I made attempts to be inclusive of women of different ages and racial and ethnic groups, women from different family forms (single, co-habiting, married or remarried), and different educational backgrounds, occupations, religions, incomes, and parenthood statuses. For example, I sent recruitment emails and flyers to social-media groups and listservs geared toward women of color. In analyzing my data, I took an intersectional approach that stresses the importance of recognizing that women can be members of more than one social category. *Intersectionality* highlights individuals' "multiple layers of social identity" that interact with each other to produce new forms of meaning and shape social experiences.[99]

Table 1 provides information on the characteristics of the sample (all tables located in the Appendix). Participants are largely white (81 percent), college educated (84 percent), employed full time (81 percent), married (69 percent), have children (62 percent), and have household incomes of $100,000 or more (41 percent). I fully recognize that my results are therefore primarily based on the perceptions and experiences of women of privilege residing in a relatively affluent, mostly white community. Although I did not ask about gender and sexual identity, the vast majority of women could be discerned to be cisgender (i.e., identify as a heterosexual woman), as husbands and partners were referred to as "he" or "him" and recruitment materials asked for "women." Still, this is an important group of women to understand. College-educated, middle-class, white women have experienced a greater increase in alcohol use in recent years than any other group of women or men.

The participants in my sample are diverse in different ways. They are representative of women at different stages of the lifecourse, and range in age from twenty-five to sixty-eight. About a third are single and/or have no children. Among those who have children, almost one-quarter (24 percent) have children who reside with them only part of the time or are empty nesters. They are engaged in a range of occupations from teaching to public relations to sales. The women reported various religious affiliations and levels of religious involvement. Sixteen percent of the sample is Catholic, 25 percent is Protestant, 16 percent reported some other religion, and 44 percent reported no religion. Religious service attendance ranged from not attending at all (38 percent) to attending weekly (19 percent). Nearly three-quarters (72 percent) of the women considered themselves a "spiritual person." Sixty percent of the sample reported household incomes below $100,000.

Table 2 shows participants' levels of alcohol consumption. Given the topic of the study, I expected heavier-than-average drinking. Assuming participants were honest about their drinking—and I have no reason to believe that they were not based on my interactions with them—this was not the case. Most could be defined as light to moderate drinkers. During the last twelve months prior to the interview, 13 percent said they drank less than once a month and 19 percent said they drank one to three times per month. The majority drank at least weekly, with 38 percent drinking once or twice a week and 32 percent drinking three or more times a week. On a typical drinking day, 47 percent said they had just one drink, 31 percent said they had two drinks, and 22 percent said they had three or more drinks. Regarding "binge drinking" (drinking four or more drinks within a two-hour period), 47 percent of women reported not having done this in the past year, 34 percent said they engaged in binge drinking one to eleven times, and 19 percent reported having engaged in binge drinking once a month or more.

Half of the women reported having had their first drink of alcohol in their teens (age thirteen to eighteen) and before being legally allowed to drink, which matches national figures.[100] Subsequent interviews revealed that women who reported their first drink before their teens took the question to mean their first "sip" of alcohol, rather than the onset of their drinking trajectory. The majority of women reported having relatives whom they considered to be "problem drinkers." The largest group (49 percent) reported problem drinking among extended family members (aunts, cousins, grandparents, etc.), 17 percent reported problem drinking in their immediate family (parents or siblings), 19 percent reported problem drinking in both their immediate and extended family, and 19 percent reported they had no problem drinkers in the family.

Finally, participants answered a series of questions assessing the presence of an alcohol use disorder. These criteria can be found in Table 3. These figures suggest that some participants may have trouble with alcohol. Over half of the women in the study (60 percent) reported behaviors consistent with an AUD. Forty-seven percent reported AUD symptoms that are considered "mild" (two to three symptoms); 13 percent of women reported symptoms consistent with a "moderate" disorder (four to five symptoms). No women reported enough symptoms to indicate a "severe" AUD, and 41 percent reported no symptoms at all. These figures are not inconsistent with national data on the prevalence of AUDs among women discussed previously.

PLAN OF THE BOOK

Chapter 1 provides a summary of statistics and trends regarding women's drinking behavior, a review of academic studies that have investigated factors underlying women's drinking patterns, a discussion of the theoretical perspectives used to frame the study, and a description of the methodologies employed to gather the data. In chapter 2, I evaluate the applicability of established paradigms for understanding alcohol use to women and their perceptions of alcohol in relation to societal-level norms, values, and concepts.

In chapter 3, I report on participants' understandings of the intergenerational transmission of alcohol, cultural differences in their perceptions of alcohol, and their attitudes toward marijuana (which emerged as a key topic). In chapter 4, I discuss participants' views of how alcohol is portrayed in advertising, television, movies, and social media, specifically in relation to women. I asked women about the use of alcohol in various social contexts such as the workplace, and about their perceptions of "women who drink" and stigmatization. Chapter 5 focuses on alcohol in relation to motherhood and specifically women's understandings of "wine mom culture." In chapter 6, I explore how women are affected by *others'* use of alcohol. Chapter 7 provides a summary of my overall findings, implications for theory and future research, emerging alcohol reduction movements, and public policies that could shape drinking behavior. The limitations of the study are also discussed.

My goal with this book is to provide greater insight into societal forces affecting women's relationship with alcohol, their growing use of it, and its consequences for women, families, and society at large. Another of my goals is to raise societal awareness that despite gains in women's education, employment, and overall human rights (including "the right to drink"), stigma against women's use of alcohol remains, forcing women to walk a very thin line, as with most features of their lives (as workers, mothers, and sexual beings), regarding what, where, when, and how much they drink. This is also a study of women for their own sake, not simply in relation to men and what men think and do. I hope the stories presented here provide comfort and reassurance to women if they are struggling with alcohol or have loved ones who are. Finally, and most importantly, this is not at all intended to be an indictment of women who drink or alcohol use in general, as is often the case in published materials. Alcohol is not, in and of itself, "bad." Most people who drink do so safely (and happily). Rather, it is an effort to understand how U.S. women navigate life in a culture that encourages the widespread consumption of alcohol. Arguably, they are navigating life so well their increasing reliance on alcohol has gone largely unnoticed. The first thing I did was ask participants what comes to mind when they think about alcohol. Although they seemed struck by the simplicity of the question, what they said was interesting, insightful, and greatly contributes to our understandings of theories, language, norms, and values surrounding alcohol from the perspective of women. This is the subject of chapter 2.

Chapter Two

Beneath the Surface

SUSAN: What does the phrase "social drinker" mean to you?

ZOEY: I always find that interesting, because if you ask, 99 percent of people will say they drink socially, but when you ask amounts, that could be from one time a year to every single social situation. Like, I drank the whole entire time, but since I'm out socializing, it's social drinking, you know?

—Zoey, age 48, therapist

Americans' attitudes toward alcohol have ebbed and flowed since the Colonial era, but it remains "a pervasive and deep-rooted feature of American life."[1] To get a baseline picture of the role of alcohol in women's lives and its meaning to women, I thought it first important to evaluate the usefulness of established paradigms and approaches to understanding alcohol consumption. Toward this end, I asked participants about their perceptions of alcohol and drinking in relation to societal-level norms, values, and concepts. (It is important to emphasize once again that the thoughts and feelings of the participants in my study are not representative of all women, especially women of color and those with less education and income. However, the in-depth information I gathered on these topics can provide a deeper level of insight into women's motivations to drink alcohol and their behavior within the broader social context than can other methodologies.) Also in this chapter, I introduce the women who participated in the study and describe their basic demographic characteristics, including their age, relationship status, and occupation. Chapter 5 focuses specifically on the perceptions of women with children.

PERCEPTIONS, CONCEPTS, DEFINITIONS

At the beginning of each interview, I asked participants their general thoughts on alcohol. *When you think about alcohol and drinking, what kinds of words and images come to mind?* Participants' initial responses reflect Americans' longstanding beliefs about alcohol in that they viewed alcohol and drinking in a rigid and polarized way.[2] A third of participants (34 percent) only described alcohol in positive terms, using words such as "good times," "celebration," "relax," and "social." Ginny, a twenty-six-year-old, married graduate student, said, "[I think of] like, friends, playing pool. Being outside. Campfires. That kind of stuff, I guess." Similarly, Olivia, a fifty-four-year-old, single project manager, said, "Great dinners, you know, good food, friends. Just hanging out with friends," and Christine, a thirty-nine-year-old, single communications specialist, responded, "What immediately popped to mind was a nice dinner and it's low lit. And there are two beautiful mixed drinks on a table, and it's part of that eating out with somebody that you enjoy and experience."

A somewhat smaller number of participants (22 percent) saw alcohol and drinking in solely negative terms, using words such as "troublesome," "dangerous," "rehab," and "alcoholic." These participants noted family members who have trouble with alcohol, health risks, and drunk driving. Joellyn, a forty-year-old, married teacher, said, "There's something funny about the word alcohol that makes my mind automatically go to alcoholic." Lori is a thirty-year-old, married human services director. She responded, "Not good things, I guess. Just like, it's been a problem in my family." Only two participants saw alcohol in what can be considered neutral terms. Janet, a twenty-eight-year-old, married bartender, said, "Just kind of like, thinking about my job, science, actually. The science behind the drink. Making it. The design of the cocktail. The quality of the cocktail. The quantity of the ingredients in the cocktail." Zoey, who was quoted previously, replied, "I guess my mind goes to advertising for some reason. When you say that, I think about all the advertising there is for different kinds of alcohol. So, in my brain, I'm seeing the Clydesdale horses or whatever."

Recall I had not asked respondents to specifically describe "positive" and "negative" aspects of alcohol. I asked them to simply talk about what comes to mind. Even respondents who saw more than one side to drinking (38 percent) discussed alcohol in opposing ways, as either "good" or "bad." As Hannah, a thirty-one-year-old, married therapist, said, "A party. Time with friends, and then I guess you get into the negative stuff like alcoholism and things like that, like liver disease. So, I guess both the positives and negatives." Jan, a thirty-year-old, married graduate student, responded, "I think I associate it in my mind as a bit of a treat, like, oh that's something fun that you do as a treat. I think there are definitely negative sides to drinking too, so that probably pops in as well. Different misuse issues and problems it can cause in society and stuff like that." Nadine, a single, forty-six-year-old human services professional, said, "It's tailgating. It's my thing. Yeah. So, that's for the most part, and then usually a kind of negative connotation I have is my stepdad drinks a lot and kind of affects, like, family functions and dynamics and stuff." However, the ability of some participants (still the minority) to view alcohol from multiple angles simultaneously is consistent with public attitudes, which as noted in chapter 1 are ambivalent, with a high level of acceptance alongside a high level of concern.[3]

Granted, a limiting factor in participants' responses is that the list of words available in our everyday language to describe alcohol use is short and contributes to the polarization in attitudes ("abstainer" and "social drinker" versus "binge drinker" and "alcoholic"). Slang is heavily skewed toward drunkenness and problem drinking (e.g., "trashed," "smashed," "bombed"), and scientific terminology is awkward and would probably be met with puzzled looks (e.g., "My friend Donna has an alcohol use disorder"). Only binge drinking is measured in a standardized way by researchers (typically five or more drinks in a two-hour period for men; four or more drinks for women), although some have questioned the validity of this measure, especially for women whose response to alcohol is more variable.[4] Otherwise, researchers conceptualize alcohol consumption in quantitative terms using a combination of frequency (e.g., number of days) and volume (e.g., number of drinks consumed), or measure alcohol consumption as a matter of degree: light, moderate, heavy. Common vernacular like *abstinence, social drinking, alcoholic,* and *binge drinking* provide somewhat more context: where consumed, what consumed, when consumed, with whom consumed, and assumptions about the drinker's (or non-drinker's) motivations, feelings, and consequences. Such measures are valuable, especially in relation to the average person's understanding of heavy drinking's association with serious health consequences. I thought exploring these concepts with participants could shed light on women's drinking behavior and yield information that conventional measures of consumption cannot.

Abstinence

After gathering participants' initial impressions of alcohol, I asked them to define a series of terms. When it comes to abstinence, responses indicated that it is not *drinking* that requires explanation, but *not drinking* (a theme throughout subsequent chapters). As Vera, a twenty-six-year-old, single public relations professional, said, "That's a good question, you know, I haven't actually thought about that. I think, to me, my initial perception is, 'Oh, that's kind of odd.' That may be because alcohol is a part of our social habits, right?" Participants, all of whom must drink at least occasionally to be included in the study, did not know very many abstainers, suggesting that drinkers are embedded in families, friendship networks, and communities with other drinkers. Tabitha, a thirty-year-old, married legal assistant, said of a friend, "I knew her for a couple of years while she wasn't drinking, but I think she's the only person I know that completely doesn't anymore." One would think defining *abstinence* would be straightforward (i.e., a person who does not drink) but that was not the case. Zoey did not see abstinence as an absolute. "I mean, I know people. I have a really good friend who is very . . . I mean it's not that she *never*, *ever* would drink, but she doesn't. Every once in a while, she likes mimosas, and maybe a couple of times a year she'll go to brunch and tell her husband, you have to drive, because I'm gonna drink a couple of mimosas, you know?" Even researchers are beginning to challenge the "no alcohol" policy on abstaining. Alcohol researcher William Kerr and colleagues examined the implications of using a more relaxed definition of abstention that expands abstaining beyond *current* abstainers, which is highly selective of people who used to drink but stopped due to health problems.[5] They created categories of abstention, ranging from "lifetime abstainers" to "lifetime minimal drinkers" to "occasional drinking."

Along with providing looser definitions of abstaining than anticipated, many participants made assumptions about the overall lives of people who abstain from alcohol (e.g., "Are you abstaining from other things in life as well? Is there a reason why you're abstaining?") and attached motivations for not drinking, such as a person's religion forbids it, their family doesn't drink, or they have had problems with alcohol. Ava, a single, twenty-five-year-old IT consultant, explained, "I'm originally from Texas and we're a big church family. So there's quite a few people with no alcohol in the house at all. Barbecues are alcohol free." Although abstaining from alcohol was questioned, it was viewed relatively positively. Bonnie, a forty-five-year-old, married massage therapist, said, "Think that's a character quality. Some of them, I think, might have had someone in their life who abused it, and that's why they are [abstaining]. I think there's a reason behind the abstaining. But it's still a quality choice."

Social Drinker

A Google Scholar search indicates there is no definitive definition of the popular term "social drinker" in the scientific literature. Given its widespread usage (for example, it is a common sorting mechanism on dating apps), it is surprising the term appears so infrequently. A *Psychology Today* article defines a social drinker simply as "individuals who drink in low-risk patterns," which the author equates to the NIAAA definition of "low-risk," which they define as no more than seven drinks per week and no more than three drinks per sitting for females and fourteen drinks per week and no more than four drinks per sitting for males.[6] Given the prevalence of the word "social drinker" in everyday language, I sought greater clarity and asked my participants to define a social drinker. Based on their responses, social drinking is comprised of six key components: it occurs *outside the home, with friends*, happens *only occasionally*, involves a *minimal amount of alcohol*, is *not the main focus* of the activity, and is *not a problem*. Typical responses were "To me that means that you drink with your friends. You drink with people. You drink when there's something going on. When there's some kind of activity," and, "Being with more people than just yourself. I consider myself a social drinker. I would say as long as you're not by yourself that would be social drinking." Leigh is a thirty-seven-year-old, married professor. She said, "If someone tells me they're a social drinker, I would assume that they do not have a drink every day at home. For me, it's like, okay, this person will be drinking when they're out and about with their friends." Participants also placed a limit on the amount: "one to two tops" and "a glass of wine or a beer." Social drinkers were seen to drink sporadically, and mostly outside the home: "Somebody who maybe has a drink with dinner sometimes, maybe like in a social setting at a party, that type of thing, like an after-work party, or work get-together, that type of thing."

All the participants considered themselves social drinkers. Yet, their reports of their own drinking were not always consistent with the "one to two drinks out with friends" rule. In the survey portion of the study, nearly a quarter of participants (22 percent) reported drinking three or more drinks on a typical day when they drank. Forty percent of participants said they did this three or more times a week. And are they really just drinking in the company of others outside the home? A higher percentage of U.S. alcohol consumers drink inside the home than outside (90 percent versus 77 percent). Twice the amount of alcohol is consumed at home as in restaurants and bars.[7] Nevertheless, my participants were adamant that social drinking only occurs outside the home, and if at home, with other people. But is this a realistic? For example, roughly half (48 percent) of U.S. women (and 31 percent of my participants) are unmarried, and single-person households still make up over one-quarter (28 percent) of all U.S. households.[8] Among singles, dating apps, FaceTime, and Zoom provide alternatives to the "bar scene," and on-demand video services such as Amazon, Netflix, and Apple TV have shifted entertainment to the home. And how common is girls' night, really? Women, especially mothers, have little time to go out. Nevertheless, the possibility that women would drink in their home on their own introduced confusion to participants. Melanie, a sixty-eight-year-old, married administrative assistant, said, "I define [social drinking] as someone who is in a social setting and they have a drink or two. Social to me is someone who does not drink at home alone. Then again, you can have . . . well maybe not. You could have a drink at home and be social." In the end, though, she says, "But to me it's like a drink or two, relaxing, socializing, kind of fitting in, that's it." Jan had trouble articulating her thoughts:

> JAN: I would define a social drinker as someone who generally drinks in the company of others, but not on their own, so they drink because it's a way to connect with other people. If someone says they're a social drinker, I would sort of put an exclusion there that they can't. I wouldn't apply that term to someone who drinks, like, on their own, or when they're by themselves, or at home as much.
>
> SUSAN: Do you have a name for that behavior?
>
> JAN: Oh! Like, a non-social drinker? Like it's the opposite? [laughs]. Um, I . . . hmm . . . in my mind I would say that they're drinking to fulfill something else in themselves as opposed to a social connection so I would maybe call that . . . I'm not sure I would call that a *lonely* drinker, because they may not be lonely, but it's that idea that there's something that they're using drinking to fulfill innately in themselves.

The vast majority of participants saw social drinking as the only acceptable context for drinking and were at a loss as to what to call drinking that was not that. Participants associated drinking on one's own at home or at a bar with sadness or problem drinking. Vera said, "In the back of my mind, social drinking versus being at home, drinking a six pack all by yourself, alone in a house, I'd be much more worried about the person. It would instill some worry in me that somebody is alone drinking much more than if somebody goes out and gets sloshed with their friends." Similarly, Isabel, a twenty-six-year-old, married researcher, said, "So, like, if you're a social drinker in my mind you're somebody who is probably not home drinking by yourself. You're drinking when you're out with people. Out for dinner. Going out. You're not like depending on alcohol when you get home at the end of the day and you're sitting on your couch." Only Janet, the bartender, came close to challenging this perception, "At a bar sometimes there's somebody drinking alone and sometimes it seems sad. Like you want to feel sad, so intuitively, like, that's so sad, but also you don't know. You don't know what's going on. They could be just, like, got off work. Like, I go to the bar sometimes after work and sit down, veg out, get my planner and my to-do list, and rectify all the pieces of paper accumulating in my bag."

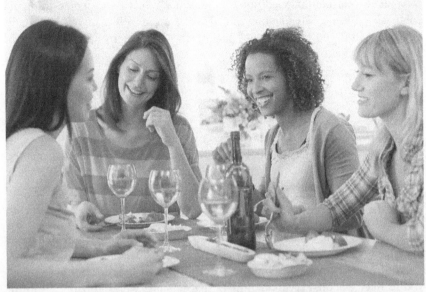

All my participants considered themselves "social drinkers," even in the face of behavior suggesting otherwise. *Source*: MBI/Alamy Stock Photo, Image ID: E3JTR1

Participants also saw social drinking as non-problematic (aside from Zoey, mentioned at the beginning of the chapter). Megan is a fifty-one-year-old, single marketing director. She said, "To me, a social drinker is somebody that enjoys a glass of wine. When they're out with friends, maybe has a glass of wine with dinner at home, but somebody that doesn't get drunk all the time, but just enjoys it. Moderately." Olivia defined a social drinker as, "somebody who is going to have one to two drinks out with friends, usually dinner is involved. Not somebody who's going to drink to an extreme where you're consuming enough alcohol that you really don't want them driving or walking down the street by themselves." And Jennifer, a thirty-three-year-old, married stay-at-home mom, said, "I guess probably someone who would prefer to have a drink in their hand, but doesn't get completely blitzed." Ella, a forty-four-year-old, married health-care provider, described it this way: "A social drinker is somebody who, if they're at dinner, drinks with a friend . . . they'll have a drink or two. When I think of social drinker, it doesn't come as a *problem*, right? That doesn't equal the same thing." Ginny's comments echo those of others: "It's part of a social situation. It's not like, let's go get *wrecked*. It'd be like, oh, let's go *casually* have a beer or two or talk about whatever thing we want to talk about and just catch up in general and do it in a social setting, like, go out to a place." Overall, participants were suspicious of any drinking not considered social. Like Brenda, a forty-three-year-old, married nurse. She said, "When I see people using alcohol a lot I think, what's going on? There's more to it than you just really enjoy it. And if you're the type of person who *really* enjoys it, a "drinker" in my lexology, there's something going on."

BINGE DRINKING

Participants considered binge drinking a wholly separate activity than social drinking. Aside from high school and college, none of the women volunteered that they currently engaged in this behavior. Yet, on the survey, more than half the participants reported alcohol consumption that met the criteria for binge drinking one to eleven times within the past year, with one in five having done so monthly or even more frequently. Only one participant raised the possibility, without my first asking, that social drinking might involve more than just one or two drinks, albeit unintentionally. That was Ginny, who said, "If you're having a really good time, you might get a second bottle and then you're like, whoops!" Although many participants were probably aware of the "official" definition of binge drinking, none used it, preferring "somebody who drinks to excess," "the purpose of it is to get drunk," "drinking a whole bunch of drinks all at once until inebriated." Most definitions included factors in addition to volume: who, where, when, and why. Two groups of binge drinkers were identified. The first was *college students* who drink *outside the home* in order to *release steam*. Sandra, a twenty-six-year-old, single teacher, said, "I think of a college-type setting where you just try to see how much alcohol you cram in before it all comes back out [laughter]. When I started college, I did the usual jungle juice, throw up all night, and not drink for a week, but what I would consider normal, freshman college experience."

When asked what comes to mind when she hears "binge drinking," Ginny said, "Oh, like college house parties. And like going on a rager or bar crawl and just being like, 'We're going out.' I feel like when people say, 'We're going out,' that's, like, someone's getting shit-faced." Participants' focus on college days corresponds to scientific literature on women's alcohol use, which is dominated by studies of college students and young adults. Most participants did not judge this type of binge drinking negatively or speculate on the reason; the desire to "party" was sufficient motivation. The majority of participants discussed how they engaged in binge drinking at one time. Like Hannah: "If I think about times in my life where I've [binge drank], I think of, like, college. Binge drinking was probably fairly prevalent in my life." Even younger women distanced themselves from this behavior as "a long time ago" (see "othering" in chapter 6). Most stories of binge drinking were not fond memories. Rather, they were told in terms of a phase best forgotten. An example is Bonnie:

> BONNIE: I remember when I was fresh out of high school and I had moved [to a different city]. For whatever reason. I don't know. I don't. I don't know if I was searching for something that I wasn't getting. And this was the only way that I knew to get it. Whoever was hosting, they had the alcohol there. And I ended up sleeping with just a random guy. And it's like, I don't even understand why. But it's, like, just scary to think that so much more could have happened.
>
> SUSAN: When you think back, were you scared at the time?
>
> BONNIE: No. I was just . . . I felt kind of oblivious to even what was going on, which wasn't really smart by any means.

Participants identified another type of binge drinker: one that *has issues* and is *out of control*. They assigned a completely different set of motivations for binge drinking outside the college context among older adults. "I see some people that are just in it for the partying. But then there's the other side where you've got the alcoholic where they have to have that drink. It's got to be there and it's totally disrupting their life." "I think there's, like, much more, like, you drink to kind of get away from feelings kind of thing. I think that's more kind of coping with something." "Problems, potentially in trouble, potentially having issues with their jobs or families, relationships. Out of control." Many participants equated binge drinking with a lack of control.

> JAN: I would say someone who drinks copious amounts of alcohol, in terms of their getting some type of strong physical or mental response, so, like, throwing up, or just severely impaired even if you don't throw up, or passing out, something like that. I also get this impression of something that's not controlled. But it's almost an involuntary thing that once you start you can't really stop.

Olivia's response was similar: "I see it as somebody who's going to go out and there's not much control to their drinking. Once they start, they don't stop until they're either broke or falling down or whatever they're drinking is empty." Unlike college binge drinking, this type of binge drinking was seen as interfering with relationships. According to Vera, binge drinking is "as many drinks as it takes for your core attitudes and your core treatment of other people to shift." Participants judged this behavior negatively. Lori said, "I picture someone who's, like, sick and not making good choices."

In the end, participants did not see much overlap between social drinking and binge drinking and did not entertain the possibility of other patterns of drinking (aside from alcoholism). When I asked, Isabel said, "I don't know if I ever put them together, but I could see if, like, you're a social drinker, you're going out with your friends, you could binge while you're out with friends. But I think I've always thought of it more of like a girls' night or a date night." Many participants in the study reported drinking more than what the Dietary Guidelines for Americans considers "healthy" for women (i.e., one drink or less per day) and 60 percent reported behaviors consistent with a mild or moderate AUD.[9] I asked participants directly about this: *I'm wondering about that space between social drinker and alcoholic. How would you define that or what would you call that?* This question was most often followed by a long pause and "I don't know," "I don't have a name for that," and "That's a good point." Nadine was one of the few women who had thought about this: "You know, I know a lot of people who gradually creeped through that space based on, like, life and stress and things like that. I've seen a good friend of mine that went through a divorce who I would say rarely drank and just kind of gradually increased to take the edge off. She kind of stopped herself before it was becoming a problem."

Alcoholic

Like social drinking and binge drinking, participants' definitions of alcoholic contained some key components: it is a *long-term* disorder, alcoholics drink *continuously* and drink mostly *alone*, alcoholics are *dependent* on alcohol, and alcoholism has *dire consequences*. Participants' comments included, "I feel like that's drinking all the time, every night, and starts interfering with work and whatnot." "Where they *have* to have that drink. It's got to be there and it's totally disrupting their life." "It comes first over family or their job, and first over them making a rational decision on anything else that matters." "Someone who probably drinks every day? Probably when they wake up to when they go to bed." "When you have to a drink every day and cannot function without having it, you know? You crave it and you have to have it, and if something tries to stop you from having it then you're just grouchy and miserable until you have it, I guess." Their definitions of alcoholism largely matched many of the items in the DSM-5's criteria for an alcohol use disorder (see Table 3).

Participants were overall sympathetic toward alcoholics and felt that alcoholism arose from a complex set of genetic, family, and situational factors including poor mental health, periods of crisis, chronic stress, childhood neglect and trauma, and an overall lack of social and emotional support. Many saw alcoholism as a form of addictive behavior not unlike overeating or gambling. As Olivia stated: "Alcoholism is like any other addiction, and there's all sorts of different studies and everything else out there, but some say there's a genetic disposition towards addiction of one form or another, whether it's alcohol or adrenaline or chocolate." Sela, a thirty-nine-year-old, married sales manager, said, "I think that many alcoholics need something, whether it's alcohol, whether it's drugs, whether it's food, whatever, it might be sex too." To Tabitha, alcoholism is "a lack of self-control during a certain period of your life, whether you have, like, some depression or something else going on. You turned to alcohol and then it just escalates. And then I could see that'd be really hard to turn off."

Most women mentioned poor mental health or an unsupportive or abusive childhood as factors. Ava describes her aunt, who passed away alone at home from an alcohol overdose: "I think there was a lot of kind of mental illness going on with her. She was always causing trouble. I guess anytime she babysat, she'd, like, lock my mom and her sister outside of the house and threaten them if they came in. She was, like, always crazy . . . not *crazy* but something wasn't right." Hannah talked about her father:

> HANNAH: I think that my dad has the kind of insecure personality where he would need to have drinks to feel like he had anything to contribute to the conversation or something like that, and maybe his [lack of] confidence? I know that maybe his dad wasn't the nicest to them when they were growing up. I think there was, he's never said it, but I think there was probably some level of abuse even if it wasn't extreme. And so I think that childhood trauma and things like that can lead to self-medicating.

I asked participants how someone becomes an alcoholic. Jan said,

> JAN: I would say my best guess would be home problems. When you are a child, if you had a home that's unstable or where there's abuse or other major issues. I don't know this, but I'm betting that, having a close family member who's an alcoholic will probably influence whether you'll become an alcoholic as well. I think that a lot of poor peer groups and support systems and pivotal times, like junior high to high school. There can be triggering life events.

Hannah also described her aunt:

> HANNAH: I would say that she's having an issue with alcohol right now. She just recently went through a divorce and I think she's self-medicating. She's really struggling. My mom tells me that [my aunt] is drinking a lot when she gets home from work. I also know she's drinking too much because my cousin who just got married two weeks ago needed wine bottles for their wedding décor and my aunt was able to supply all of them that they needed! [laughs]

Some women told stories that were consistent with the conventional narrative promoted by A.A., which sees alcoholism in black-and-white terms: either you have the lifelong disease of alcoholism or you don't, with people inevitably spiraling downward into alcoholism and despair, only able to crawl out after "hitting rock bottom." Janet talked about her father-in-law: "He's an alcoholic. He hasn't drank in twenty years or something, but he calls himself an alcoholic." Yet, as discussed in chapter 1, the findings of many studies do not support the inevitable descent-into-alcoholism idea, and it's been established that alcohol usage declines with age. And counter to the "once an alcoholic, always an alcoholic'" mantra of A.A., a study based on the National Survey on Drug Use and Health showed that only 10 percent of heavy drinkers met the criteria for an alcohol use disorder.[10] Despite providing conventional definitions of an alcoholic, participants provided many stories of people who were heavy drinkers at one time, stopped drinking, and then resumed using alcohol (recall, too, that many participants reported they themselves engaged in heavy periods of binge drinking). Bonnie told about her nephew:

BONNIE: He had tendencies with drugs and alcohol, even in high school. He would drink *so* much. He would get to the point where he'd either pass out or throw up and then keep drinking. But when you get pulled over for just a random traffic stop and you're still drunk the next morning, that's a problem. So he spent probably five or six years in A.A. And then realized that he had control and then started adding alcohol back into his life just because he wanted to. And we all just kind of took a step back and . . . it's like you hold your breath to see how it pans out. And he's done well. He's done very well.

Brenda talks about her mother:

BRENDA: Me and the kids would go over to do something and she was drunk and I would say to her, go back in the house. I don't want the kids to see it. Do not come back out. I mean, she couldn't walk straight. It was like five o'clock at night. She's been drinking all day. She's complained that the eye doctor didn't give her the right prescription for her glasses. I think that was playing a huge role in her feeling, like, worthless, and not able to do things she wanted to do. [Since she got new glasses] she's back to sewing, she's back to doing the things that she enjoys doing. And I think *that's* filling her time, and not the drinking.

Diane, a twenty-nine-year-old, married graduate student, also talked about her mom, who lost her own mother and husband in short order:

DIANE: She wasn't one to go out with her friends and have drinks. But it was when my dad had passed. Well, first her mom had passed and I noticed she had some hang-ups with alcohol, like drinking by herself and then acting drunk when I wouldn't expect her to. And then she got better. My dad got diagnosed with cancer and she had to be his caretaker. And as far as I could tell, functionally, she had gotten better. Then after he died and she stopped being his caretaker, she just deteriorated really quickly. It's been about three years now. An episode where she'll just drink to oblivion is a lot less frequent than when he just passed. But she'll still have a drink every now and then.

Like people's ability to move in and out of heavy drinking, the notion of a "functional alcoholic" presents a problem to conventional narratives, as does "people who don't know they are an alcoholic." Christine's description of her brother-in-law strayed into this gray area:

CHRISTINE: Sometimes it's hard to tell from the outside. He does not reach the bar on any of those. I mean, he's been a successful parent of his own daughter, goes to work every day. Like, I don't notice anything that seems like he's interfering with his life. He certainly drinks more than I did when I was growing up. I still feel fine about him. If I thought it was a problem, I wouldn't want him around my son.

Melanie put alcoholics into two categories:

MELANIE: There's the type that they're aggressive. They get into trouble. They may miss work and they'll get sick, that kind of alcoholic. But then I've known men that are definitely alcoholics that went to work every day and never missed a day. As soon as they got home, they were drinking, but they never missed a day. And they worked like that for years. To me, that's a functioning alcoholic.

SUSAN: Do you think they would consider themselves alcoholics?

MELANIE: No, I know they didn't.

Megan's story of a good friend runs counter to the idea that people who drink a lot can't control themselves:

SUSAN: Does [your friend] think she has an issue with alcohol?

MEGAN: She does. She's tried some of the medications to keep you from drinking. She's tried to give it up altogether. I haven't asked her recently where she's at with it, but I get the impression that she's still drinking. But it ebbs and flows for her. Sometimes she can be "good" and have one or two drinks. And other times she can finish a bottle, and she doesn't drink when she goes out because she has to drive herself.

That heavy drinkers sometimes test themselves to "see if they're an alcoholic" also challenges the disease model of alcoholism. Cindy, a fifty-four-year-old, single research coordinator, said, "After my conversation with my husband I deliberately did not have a drink the whole week until now, and so I'm like, yeah, okay. So you are not an alcoholic basically." Participants agreed that it could be difficult to determine when a person has "crossed the line" into alcoholism. As Diane said, "It comes on so gradually once you realize it, it's too late . . . I think it's probably gradual over time, like that old analogy about the frog that boils slowly in the pot." Regarding her siblings, she says:

DIANE: I think my brother and sister are getting there. I definitely think my sister's there.

SUSAN: Getting toward being an alcoholic?

DIANE: I think my sister is probably an alcoholic.

SUSAN: What makes you think that?

DIANE: Whenever I see my sister, as soon as she walks in the door, she's got a drink. She'll take it with her if we're going out to eat and she'll, like, have to bring it with her.

Jan said, "I think my husband's family are just heavier drinkers. He might say his mom is a bit of a problem drinker. I don't know. But not from my perspective. None of them are over the edge." Zoey's long and rather convoluted description of alcoholism likewise demonstrates the limitation of conventional narratives:

ZOEY: I just assessed a guy to be a kidney donor a few months ago and he absolutely is a problem drinker. Like, absolutely, 100 percent. You would probably give him an addiction diagnosis, but when I also looked at it, I mean, he can also stop on a dime. Like, he doesn't have the *physical* addiction. It's more, I felt like, more for him a habit. It's what he *does*. It works for him. He has not had negative consequences from it. Like, he goes to work every day and he's successful in his job and his relationships are good. No legal trouble from drinking. I feel like if any of those other things were different, and you have the same drinking pattern, people would look at it more as, "you're an alcoholic." Like he absolutely in my book is an alcoholic but because of those *key* things he doesn't see it as that.

Only a few participants were judgmental of alcoholics. Glenda, a twenty-nine-year-old, married daycare teacher, thought of alcoholism as a choice: "I feel like for an alcoholic you have to consciously make that decision to also keep drinking. Like maybe they're using alcohol as a coping skill or something and they don't want to try something else. Like, hey! You should try running! Nope, I'm good! Oh, okay, alrighty then! Case closed." Nadine's views were similar: "I believe it's a disease and stuff, but I also feel like people's choices get them there. I know that there's genetic things and stress and life and situational things, but I feel like nobody forces you to, like, keep putting that drink up to your lips type of thing." Others mentioned alcoholism can be dealt with through "hard work," like Jennifer, who said, "I grew up in an alcoholic home. I started doing self-help stuff and therapy in my early teens and have, like, pounded away at it the rest of my life. It's the only reason I'm not in jail right now or a drug addict or whatever."

CONCLUSION

My conversations suggest women's views on alcohol are polarized. They had trouble describing alcohol consumption in ways outside the realms of "good" drinking (abstinence, social drinking, binge drinking in college) and "bad" drinking (binge drinking outside of college, alcoholism). Unless pressed, participants drew upon existing frameworks, conventional terms, and traditional concepts to explain alcohol and drinking. For most participants, the only acceptable drinking was social drinking, which was restricted to *occasionally* having *one or two drinks* while out with *family or friends*. Not *every day*. Not home *alone*. Not the *main purpose*. And definitely *not a problem*. In fact, all the participants defined themselves as social drinkers, despite reporting alcohol usage clearly outside their own definitions. Their descriptions of an "alcoholic" were consistent with A.A., despite knowing people who did not fit this pattern. The idea that heavy drinkers might just be heavy drinkers was unpopular. Participants also made assumptions regarding drinkers' emotions, motivations, and the consequences of substance use. They were sympathetic to people they considered alcoholic or who were otherwise struggling with alcohol. In chapter 3, I explore participants' understandings of how beliefs about alcohol are internalized and transmitted across generations, and the extent to which beliefs are uniquely American. My first few conversations suggested that marijuana was an additional topic to pursue. This, combined with changing attitudes toward marijuana and the loosening legal restrictions across states, led me to routinely ask participants their feelings about the acceptability of marijuana and mood-altering substances more broadly.

Chapter Three

Changing Tides

GLENDA: I'm pro-cannabis. I actually like it better than drinking. I just feel like there's less side effects from it, if you will. Like if I smoke a blunt I'm not gonna feel like crap tomorrow and not show up for my shift, whereas if I drink a crap-ton of beer or liquor then I'm gonna feel shitty the next day unless I'm smart and hydrate. But that's a lot of water. Let's be honest.

—Glenda, age 29, married, daycare teacher

Where do our ideas about the acceptability of alcohol (and other mood-altering substances) even come from? Ecological and lifecourse theories focus on how individuals' attitudes and behavior influence others in their lives, past and present. To understand how beliefs about alcohol are transmitted among people and internalized by individuals, I asked participants to describe what they were told about alcohol in their formative years (from parents, school, etc.), and what they told, or plan to tell, their own children. As noted in chapter 1, a family history of problem drinking is associated with higher levels of alcohol use and alcohol-related problems beyond biological predispositions. Families are the main mechanism through which children learn about alcohol, whether formal discussions are had or not. Schools, the media, peers, churches also teach lessons about alcohol. As a whole, these socialization agents deliver American children mixed messages about alcohol: drinking is fun, sophisticated, and exciting, but also dangerous, scary, and, for some, immoral. Adolescents are regularly exposed to advertising, music videos, movies, and television showing drinking in an overwhelmingly positive light.[1] Such imagery, especially when integrated within social media, has been found to encourage alcohol consumption among adolescents and adults.[2] Yet, remnants of First Lady Nancy Reagan's "Just Say No" campaign of the 1980s

persist and schools continue to take a simplistic "scared straight" approach
to drugs and alcohol. Even today, many schools bring in expensive D.A.R.E.
programs and stage car accidents despite no evidence such programs do
anything to curb drinking among youth.[3] Not to say that things aren't changing. Some schools are revamping their drug and alcohol education curricula,
moving away from the expectation of absolute abstinence toward a focus on
"harm reduction" and making healthy choices.[4]

Alcohol-related messages participants discussed receiving from their parents were primarily fear-based and focused on alcoholism, drunk driving, and
sexual assault. As Hannah said, "The only thing that sticks in my mind that
my mom and I would have talked about was to be safe when you're drinking.
Have a plan of how you're getting somewhere or just stay where you are."
Isabel said, "I think they were afraid I wouldn't be able to tell when you've
reached the point where you need to stop, and my either getting black-out
drunk or ending up in a situation or at least getting really sick, that along with
the idea of getting drugged, so keep your wits about you." When she turned
twenty-one, Glenda's parents told her:

GLENDA: Make sure you watch your drink. Because somebody could, you
know, like, try to date rape you. It's basically a lot of negative associations with
alcohol and drinking. My parents also hyped it up to seem like it was this big,
bad, terrible thing that, like, once you start doing it, it's *awful*, you're, you're
gonna downward spiral to like alcoholism and all this stuff. A lot of "nothing
good happens after midnight." But I had a glass of it and I was like, okay?
[shrugs] What's the big deal? I don't get it.

Vera's parents saw using alcohol underage as a moral failing: "It was much
less an aversion to alcohol than it was a fear of getting caught. My parents
had instilled from a very young age that if you do something wrong, you will
get caught. You will be punished. And not only that, you'll bring shame upon
our family."

Participants' discussions with their own children were softer but still
focused on danger. Melanie said in relation to her now thirty-six-year-old
daughter: "I did not scold her. I didn't feel the need to do that. She's always
been responsible. But as a female, you have to be careful how much you
drink, where you drink, how you drink, and who you drink with, all of that."
Bonnie has three teenagers. "I would just hope to God that they're smart
about their choice or have somebody there that is going to watch their back.
If you go to a party, take your own container. Keep the cap on. Don't accept
a drink from anybody. It's just not what it used to be. It's not the days when
you fill the bathtub with whatever and scoop some out." Sela talks about her
seventeen-year-old son: "He informed me just a couple months ago that he

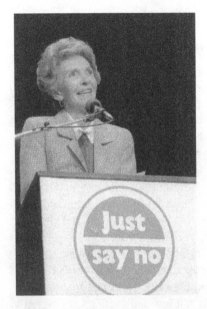

Former First Lady Nancy Reagan's "Just Say No" campaign of the 1980s was ineffective in curbing drug and alcohol use in children. *Source*: National Archives Catalog, https://catalog.archives.gov/id/75855449

tried vodka and he likes vodka. And I was like, oh, okay. I said, you know, your grandpa and your aunt have problems with alcohol, and understand that that's something that could potentially be in you as well."

BURYING THE PAST?

It makes sense that participants' past experiences influenced what they told their own kids. There were many stories of bad hangovers. But also more serious situations such as having to drive people to the hospital after an alcohol overdose, saving girlfriends from sexual predators, blacking out, and worries about alcohol dependence. Isabel says about her time in college: "I was getting to a point when I did get black-out drunk a couple times and then it was that shame the next day of not knowing what I had said, what I had done. That was excruciating." Olivia said, "I realized by my senior year that I had a bit of a problem trying to cope with everything, because I was drinking a lot. I was drinking sometimes to go to bed at night, and I was drinking sometimes first thing in the morning, like a screwdriver before I went to class." There were a number of stories of near misses:

MEGAN: I was lucky, I guess you could say, in college. I mean, I definitely did things I regret. At one point I was at a fraternity house and the guys were hanging me out a third-story window by my ankles. I can remember I've driven drunk before. I've definitely had a one-night stand when I was drunk.

SUSAN: Do you think you would have slept with that person if you had not been drinking?

MEGAN: Mmm, I don't know, probably not.

That is not to say that participants didn't identify positive aspects of drinking. Participants all identified as drinkers and saw drinking as a mostly pleasurable activity. Alcohol enabled them to "relax," "let their hair down," and "let loose" with friends. Participants saw alcohol as a kind of "social lubricant" that enhances fun and reduces anxiety in awkward situations such as meeting new people. Jennifer thought back to her college days: "It wasn't like an everyday thing, but I did drink a lot then. I'm not gonna lie to you. Okay? I had a blast, you know, probably Friday or Thursday through Saturday. Like most college kids, I would over-drink and barf my brains out and just did the stupid regular college thing. And then, you know, your studies get more intense, so you just, like, pull it together, right?" Kim is twenty-eight, married, and works in health care. She also describes positive experiences: "It was at someone's house, and we'd play some games. Nothing too crazy. We just had more fun playing the games and talking and stuff so we weren't *drinking*. It was social drinking but nothing *crazy*. Not college-style parties like I had been to." A number of women said that they liked to try different kinds of cocktails and that it enhances the taste of food. Glenda explained, "If I have a steak, I like to have a shiraz with it to balance the steak. I pair my stuff. If we have fish, we have a white wine to go with it. Not all the time but sometimes. If it's burgers, we'll have beer."

I learned that participants who had talked to their children about alcohol for the most part omitted their own drinking history. Some were concerned

RHYMES WITH ORANGE   **BY HILARY B. PRICE**

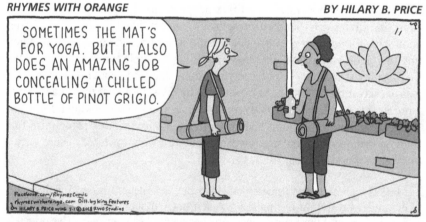

Source: Rhymes With Orange © 2018 RWO Studios, Dist. by King Features Syndicate, Inc.

that admitting they drank to excess themselves somehow diminished their authority on the subject. Like Ella: "My husband really didn't drink in high school. He didn't drink until he got to college. His freshman year he went nuts. He will admit that. But we could both say to them with a straight face we did not drink in high school." Rather than using their own experiences, participants generalized risks and focused on helping their children make "good choices" and develop skills to navigate social encounters that involve alcohol. Cindy explained, "I've talked to my daughter about responsible drinking, you know, preserve your brain and wait until you're twenty-six and you're done growing." Jan, who did not have children, said, "I want to take the approach that essentially my parents took. Which is not laying a taboo on X, Y, and Z, but tending to things like helping children have goals in life. Be involved in multiple things, in multiple areas. Getting them in a positive peer group. With these, I feel like the desire or need for these other things lessens." Participants made more of an effort than their own parents to provide their children with skills and tools. Brenda, a nurse, said, "I talk with my kids pretty openly about drinking and drugs and that sort of stuff and I give them real life examples of things I've seen and if something comes up I'll say, okay, so this is what I saw at work today. What do you guys think about that? What would you do?"

ALCOHOL POLICE

And how are these messages received? Many studies indicate that children have both positive and negative feelings toward alcohol and are more ambivalent about drinking than they are about other substances.[5] For reasons not fully known, but likely having to do with social media and having fewer in-person interactions, Gen Z and millennials are drinking significantly less than previous generations did at their age.[6] Brenda speculates, "I wonder if that's because they're learning about the dangers of alcohol and whatnot, and they want their parents to be safe and that's kind of the reason behind it much more than their judging them." A number of women even described being "policed" by their children. Lori has two children, ages seven and ten. "They see us, like, drink a glass of wine or whatever. They like are getting the messaging in school because when my older son sees someone drinking beer, he's like, 'Oh, you shouldn't do that!' [laughter] So they're like, 'Mom, that's not good for you' type of thing." Sela told her kids, "'It's okay for mom and dad to have a glass of wine or a beer, but not all the time. It's not good for our body or our brains.' That's kind of as far as we went, but it's funny, the seven-year-old, every time I buy a bottle of wine at the store, he's like,

'Put that back! You don't need that!'" Cindy told a story about a trip she took with her daughter:

> CINDY: A couple of years ago, we went on one of these tours of Europe. There were sixteen retired teachers from the U.S. They were heavy drinkers *every night*. They were rowdy. They drank a lot. She somehow was traumatized by that. She would say, "These are *teachers*, why are they doing this?" It impacted her so that she didn't want to be around them. After that, if she saw me having a glass of something she'd be like, "Mom, I don't want you to lose control. Don't become like them."

Other studies have found that children keep track of the alcohol consumption of their parents. A participant in a study of low-income, urban, mostly black women who were both problem drinkers and had experienced intimate partner violence said, "I taught him. He knows what an adult beverage is, so he will even say, 'are you drinking an adult beverage?' and I'm like yeah I'm having an adult beverage, and he says well I don't want any of that."[7]

ALL IN THE FAMILY

Given that alcohol consumption is so pervasive and that most adults drink, how do parents reconcile alcohol's dangers with societal norms promoting alcohol? Many participants held the working theory that they could "head off" trouble and mitigate alcohol's risks by allowing their children to drink under their supervision. "I would rather have them drink with me, and having it be something that's controlled and safe." "If you do drink, we prefer it be here." Kim said of her parents, "They preferred I do it at home. One of those, like, okay, if you want to try it, you need to be here to do it." Some parents gave their children a small amount of alcohol at family events in an effort to model responsible drinking. "I can remember getting to be a little bit older and my mom got these wine glasses that were really small," explained Megan, "and so my brother and I would get just a splash of wine at a fancy dinner, like at Christmas dinner or something. I thought I was so grown up" [laughter]. Jan said, "I drank a few times in the family so definitely it was a 'wine with dinner' type of atmosphere. I don't think I ever had a whole drink." Another strategy was to give children a "dose" of alcohol in the hopes that they wouldn't like it. Kori, a forty-nine-year-old, married medical assistant told her children, "You're going to have some friends and some other parents that think nothing of it, but my husband had already cured them. At about the age of five or six my son wanted to taste his beer. He had a sip and he was like 'blech'" [laughter]. Isabel said her parents "were never secretive about alcohol." But she remembered in fifth grade "smelling my mom's glass of wine and thinking it smelled good and asking her if I could have a sip and she let me, knowing I was gonna spit it back out." Joellyn used this tactic. "My daughter was probably eleven or twelve as I was drinking a glass of wine and she was like, 'That smells terrible. Does it taste terrible?' And I was like, 'Well, you can taste it.' And so she tasted it. I tried to make it not like a huge forbidden, terrible thing."

In reality, numerous studies indicate that none these strategies are effective in delaying or stopping underage drinking,[8] and age at onset of alcohol use is one of the strongest predictors of alcohol disorders in adolescence and adulthood.[9] In fact, children's attitudes and "alcohol expectancies" (i.e., their anticipated pattern of drinking) develop well ahead of taking their first drink.[10] Studies show that even very young children are able to identify different types of alcohol by their smell, and alcohol is frequently part of children's play ("buying" alcohol, pretending to drink, etc.).[11] They also associate alcohol with being popular and cool.[12] Positive associations of alcohol increase with age.[13] Leigh said of her daughter, "So she was two and a half and she'll be like, 'Oh, are you having an "adult" today? [laughter] Do you want the red adult or the white adult?' So, she knows those things. And we try to be very careful about that being something positive, because we don't want her in the culture that says, 'This is really bad for you, don't do it,' but hey, you're seeing me doing it every day." Carly tells her daughter, "You know, it's mommy's drink. Coffee? Can't drink it. It's mommy's drink. I don't specifically tell her what it is or anything, but at this point, I'm not going to hide it. But I'm not sure what'll happen in the future so . . . "

Studies also show that, beyond their level of use, witnessing parents consume alcohol changes children's perceptions of its acceptability.[14]

SUSAN: How do you feel about drinking around kids?

GINNY: I don't know. It just feels weird. I'm just like, I don't want your first memory of me to be just drunk. That sounds not pleasant. Because I have a niece and nephew, and they're definitely old enough to formulate, like, memories where they're probably going to remember shit, so like yeah, I'm just like, mmm . . . no."

A number of participants expressed feeling guilty about drinking around their kids. After one particular incident, Joellyn decided she would no longer drink in front of her children. "I can remember one time putting my daughter to bed and I gave her a kiss goodnight. She's like, 'Mommy, your breath smells like wine.' And she was like three or four and I really was like, how do you recognize that? So, then I questioned. I was like, gosh, do I drink too much in front of them?" Some participants took great pains to keep their alcohol

consumption from their kids. Parker is a thirty-three-year-old, married program assistant:

> PARKER: I don't ever want her to see me out of control and so that's why I've
> always thought, if I'm going to get drunk, I need to know that she has a babysit-
> ter. I don't even like the idea of like having a babysitter who leaves if I'm drunk
> that night. I don't like the idea that I'd be hungover and not able to take care of
> her if she needs anything. When she gets older, I plan to continue to have, like,
> a beer with dinner or something like that. I don't want her to think it's evil. I
> want her to see what moderation looks like.

> SELA: We didn't feel comfortable drinking around the kids, but then it became
> a thing where we were, like, kind of like sneaking a glass of wine up to our
> room and then it felt bad. It felt really just bad. We pretty much, like, didn't
> drink for a long time. And then gradually we felt more comfortable having a
> glass of wine. And then we would talk about it and say, you know, you can be
> a responsible drinker.

Compared to what they themselves learned from their own parents, participants made a greater effort to normalize drinking and model what they felt
was appropriate drinking behavior. Christine said, "If we're having a meal
and my current partner has cooked it and has poured a glass of wine for each
of us, I hope to show that you can enjoy it as part of an experience without
consuming the rest of the bottle. Some of the more problematic parts. To
show that it doesn't seem that interesting. That it doesn't seem so forbidden."

DRINKING IN AMERICA

My conversations with participants about what they were taught about alcohol and what they intend to teach their own children led to an interesting
new topic—the extent to which Americans' beliefs about alcohol are similar
or different from those of other places. Their comments reflect Americans'
ambivalence about alcohol.

> CARLY: As a society, we're very afraid of alcohol. But it's a big source of in-
> come. And I feel so there's, like, it's taboo but it's not taboo in some ways. You
> can go in the army, enlist at eighteen, but can't drink until you're twenty-one.
> We think of alcohol [so] taboo. Over in Europe, for example, like, you go to a
> family gathering and this fifteen-year-old's drinking a little bit of wine with the
> celebration for Christmas. I don't know, it's just looked down upon more here,
> but it's also oddly celebrated in a way, like at football games. It's just it goes
> hand-in-hand that feels like . . . I don't know, it's a weird relationship [laughs].

Many participants believed that America's overall approach to alcohol was associated with greater consumption. A number of women suggested that strict laws, particularly regarding age, can backfire because it presents alcohol as "forbidden" and therefore sought after among youth. Isabel's response was typical: "I never smoked weed. And I don't really have a desire to. We have to study it more, too. But for alcohol? I think having it age at twenty-one instead of eighteen like it is in Europe actually makes it more dangerous because it's a rebellious thing." Isabel's theory is not supported by data. In actuality, the U.S. is "middle of the road" when it comes to alcohol policies and regulations, such as cost, where alcohol can be sold, where and when it can be consumed, acceptable blood alcohol levels for operating a motor vehicle, and how alcohol can be advertised. Stricter laws and policies surrounding alcohol are associated with lower alcohol consumption across countries and a higher minimum drinking age is consistently associated with less drinking.[15] Nevertheless, Olivia maintained, "It is legal to drink in Europe, but it's also normalized at a very young age where it's not the kind of drinking we do here because it's done socially around the dinner table with family. You start in your early teens. Usually it's wine mixed with water. It's not seen as something horrible." This theory doesn't work either. Americans consume *less* alcohol than in France, Spain, Germany, Australia, many Eastern European countries, and Russia (but more than in Canada, Norway, Finland, and Sweden) and have lower rates of hazardous drinking than many countries such as Canada, Ireland, and New Zealand.[16] A 2017 meta-analysis of thirteen studies showed that parental rules about alcohol reduce the risk of alcohol problems in adolescence.[17]

In general, the typical way that American children are socialized to drink reflects the polarization of alcohol as either "good" or "bad," a consistent theme throughout my interviews. Sociologist Amy Schalet interviewed roughly 150 American and Dutch parents and children for her book, *Not Under My Roof*. She found marked differences in parenting in the U.S. versus the Netherlands.[18] She argues that American parents take an "adversarial" approach in moving children toward adulthood with the feeling that "the adolescent self is not yet equipped to control the strong inner passions or peer pressures and whose potentially out of control drinking must be held in check by adult supervision." American parents desire children to establish self-sufficiency, take personal responsibility, and "cut the apron strings," and do so using a heavy hand (e.g., no drinking whatsoever under any circumstances), resulting in a lot of drama and conflict. As Kori told her two teenagers, "Remember, ultimately it's still your choice. So make good choices and as soon as you're eighteen and you leave my house and you go get in trouble, you can do stupid all by yourself. I will love you every day, but I will not bail you out." In contrast, she says, Dutch parents emphasize interdependence, which assumes that "young people can and will control their alcohol intake and place their drinking in the context of the participation in sociality."[19] Parents are in continuous consultation with their children through adulthood (e.g., "let's talk about it"). Dutch parents take the view that harsh rules will encourage children to engage in forbidden behavior (whether drinking, doing drugs, or sex) in secret.

Participants' views were not inconsistent with the adversarial approach. Despite increasing emphasis on making good choices, they told their children scary stories of overdoses, sexual assault, car accidents, and DUIs. Participants exposed to alternative drinking cultures were more reflective, like Ella, who spent many years living abroad.

> ELLA: I was in Germany and the drinking age is, like, sixteen and I was sixteen. It was my first time and all these German people were so experienced with it and I felt so under experienced. I maybe only had two or three drinks because at the time I wasn't used to anything. I remember them saying, "America is so crazy." How can you have to wait until you're twenty-one? Like, sixteen is the normal age.

Leigh is from Brazil. She said, "I think the big difference is, what's the purpose of your drinking? I think one of the big differences is we're introduced to alcohol in a family setting. So you're way beyond that once you get to college. But in America, you just maximize this whole, like, drinking to get drunk." Isabel's feelings continue along these lines: "I dated a guy from Switzerland when I was in high school and I remember them being super baffled by our binge drinking culture, especially when you hit twenty-one. Because where they're from you can start drinking when you're sixteen, seventeen, and so it's not a big deal, so kids don't. It's not a rebellious activity. Here, it's kinda like for younger people a way to stick it to their parents."

In some communities, drinking says something about one's morality. Jennifer explained:

> JENNIFER: I grew up with a lot of that super-judgy crap in the back of my brain. I lived in Georgia when I was a kid and they're very weird about drinking there. It's completely different. They have dry counties and certain times a day you can sell liquor and certain days you can't even sell liquor, but you could buy beer. Like all these weird rules. My cousin owns a fantastic restaurant and he wanted a few European tables outside. He had Baptist preachers and people come out with signs and protest in front of his restaurant.

I asked Glenda what she would say about alcohol if she were to have children.

GLENDA: I would like to approach it from a European standpoint.

SUSAN: Tell me about that.

GLENDA: It's different in Europe. In Germany, kids who are ten are drinking beer like water and it's more socially acceptable there.

SUSAN: What do you think the effect of that is on children and society to have it be so socially acceptable at younger ages?

GLENDA: I almost wished my parents *did* drink because the fact that they didn't and they hyped it up to be this big bad terrible thing almost made me want to do it *more*. Whereas in Europe, kids witness their parents, I assume, drinking a lot of the time and it's just like, "Oh, okay, Mom's having a beer. Meh." You know, it's just more *relaxed*. It doesn't have such a negative undertone.

That is not to say that they didn't see alcohol being misused outside the United States. Sandra was an exchange student in college:

SANDRA: When I was in Sweden, oh my gosh. Those people are drinking crazy amounts. And these people are from Germany, France, so many Europeans all together. They drink so much.

SUSAN: When you say they drink a lot, what does that look like? Are we talking about over the course of a night, people are drinking like ten beers or they're drinking shots? Are people, like, falling down?

SANDRA: It actually is that. People are falling down almost every single Friday night. Like needing to be carried back to their room. Drinking, like, a whole bottle of vodka between three or four people. And that's just what, like, you're supposed to do when you're young and in college. In Sweden, there's a lot of very liberal young people that had a lot of drugs. I went to one or two parties and saw so many people, like, doing lines of coke.

BREATHE EASIER

My conversations with participants about how attitudes toward alcohol may be changing over time also led to a discussion of other substances, namely marijuana. Attitudes toward marijuana have become more favorable and many states have legalized marijuana for medical and recreational use. As of 2019, thirty-six states have legalized marijuana for medical purposes and sixteen states for recreational use.[20] Almost two-thirds (65 percent) of Americans think smoking marijuana is morally acceptable, and more than two-thirds (68 percent) of Americans support the legalization of marijuana, up from 32 percent in 2009.[21] In 2019, 12 percent of Americans (15 percent of men and 9 percent of women) said they smoke marijuana versus only 7 percent in 2013.[22] Overall, Americans see alcohol and other drugs as more serious problems in their communities than marijuana.[23]

Participants' attitudes toward marijuana followed national trends. The most common response was along the lines of "I'm totally fine with people using it." This was true among women who had never used marijuana or didn't use it currently: "I don't care if someone smokes, but I personally just don't. It's just not for me." "I don't use marijuana. I did in college. Occasionally. Like twice. It makes me sick. So, I just don't do it. But, like, I don't have a problem with people that do." Isabel said, "I have never smoked weed. And I don't really have a desire to. However, I think the fact that it's classified so highly, you know, it's a felony to have it, I think is ridiculous." Christine says of herself and her husband: "We sort of joke that, like, maybe we would try it if we could get our hands on it. But it turns out nerdy parents are not the first people you think to offer it to. And we're, like, not trying that hard. I just don't know where to get it."

All the participants in the study reported knowing people who use marijuana. A smaller number said they use marijuana themselves, and most have tried it. As Joellyn explained:

> JOELLYN: I don't smoke pot anymore, but I still have friends and family members, actually, who do very moderately.
>
> SUSAN: By moderately, what does that mean?
>
> JOELLYN: I would say, like, maybe a hit or two at night. Sort of like I do with a glass of wine.

People in Cindy's friend group use marijuana pretty regularly. "My friends are in their mid-fifties to early sixties. I have a couple of girlfriends who are sixty-something and they do it as recreation like every Thursday or Friday night. They take one of these edible things in five or ten milligrams and apparently enjoy it and they're like, 'Oh you should come and do this sometime,' and I was like, well . . . '"

Insteadibles

My conversations with participants suggest that some U.S. women may be moving from drinking to marijuana. As one put it, "I call them 'insteadibles.' I often sub that for alcohol. It's helpful to take the edge off and makes me sleepy and able to relax so it's usually best done when I am planning to be in bed early to watch something or chill out." A few reasons may underlie this switch. The first is that marijuana has fewer negative side effects than alcohol, namely hangovers and weight gain. As Ginny said, "If edibles were legal,

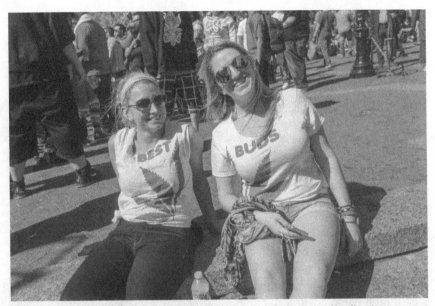

The majority of women in the United States approve of marijuana legalization. *Source*: Stacy Walsh Rosenstock/Alamy Stock Photos, Image ID ENFHJ4

I think I would probably do that more than I would drink, because I've never been hungover from weed. I think if there was an option between the two, you wanna, like, do something social, but you don't really feel like drinking." That marijuana is increasingly legal and more readily available appears to be playing a role. Parker said, "I'm excited for marijuana to be legalized. [SUSAN: Really?] Yes. I've smoked marijuana. I've done, like, edibles, mostly in Colorado where it's legal and what I like about it is that I feel fine the next day." And Ginny: "If marijuana was legal, I think I would smoke, or if I was able to get it by not smoking, because I don't actually like smoking, if edibles were legal, I think I would probably do that more than I would drink." A number of participants remarked it was less addictive than alcohol. Ginny went on to say, "I have one friend who doesn't drink because he says he's an alcoholic, because he's just like, if I start drinking I just won't stop, so he smokes weed. He probably smokes way too much weed, but that's what he does instead." Still, people are reluctant to "advertise" they use marijuana, like Sela:

SELA: I have one girlfriend here who does edibles. She has anxiety and she prefers to do that. She's like, I just take a half when I'm feeling like too much in my life, my career, my kids. I just take a half and I can just calm down. But it's a secret, like she hasn't told people. That's the way some of my friends wind down and they get up the next morning and go to work. And everything's cool. It's probably better for them than, you know, my glass of wine a couple of times a week.

Glenda was also annoyed that marijuana is seen as unacceptable, especially for women with children:

GLENDA: I do think that there is a stigma against the mom who wants the occasional glass of wine compared to the mom who needs a joint, or who wants to smoke a joint. The glass of wine is more socially acceptable. That's okay! You can do that! That's a thing! But marijuana? Oh nooo! Noooo! Nooo! It's the *gateway drug* [says in funny scary voice].

Be More Chill

Many participants noted that in addition to being less harmful to one's health, marijuana doesn't make people "act crazy" the way alcohol does. Christine, who was a resident assistant in college, explained, "I prefer to deal with people that were high rather than people that were drunk. Like, I would take a chill high person over a fighting drunk person." The legality of marijuana mattered to her. "If it was legal here, I'd get it. Being legal is important because it's public if you're arrested for something and I would worry about that professionally, and my kid knowing that even though I think those laws are dumb, it's still the law. Alcohol is an acceptable thing." Glenda and her friends smoke marijuana and said they preferred the cannabis because you get "happy and hungry." Joellyn said, "Very rarely have I ever seen anybody who is smoking marijuana get violent. More than anything else it's, you know, you sink into the couch and become one with the couch."

Janet, who suffers from chronic pain, felt the same way:

JANET: I don't think people get violent like they do on alcohol. I mean, you're, like, silly, stupid, right? I think it would be much better. I think it would probably be much better had we chosen that to be our form of relaxation, but unfortunately we chose drinking, which can really be a problem for people. A lot of it to me is just making this body feel better so I can get through functioning. I'm using it to make myself feel better so I can clean my house.

Participants overall felt that marijuana "is not like other drugs." Olivia said, "I probably would say that marijuana doesn't really concern me. Mushrooms probably don't concern me. Heroin, opiates, and all of the other stuff scare the bejesus out of me and I have no interest in trying it. I don't know anybody who uses. I feel those are true narcotics." And Glenda:

GLENDA: I feel like psychedelic shrooms and cannabis, those are their own little category or not even drugs. I don't like to call them drugs, because shrooms are natural, and marijuana is natural, and the side effects for the most part are temporary. Whereas alcohol, if you drink too much of it, your liver starts shutting down and then you need a liver transplant, or you can ruin your relationship. Like you can give alcohol to someone who's never been angry before in their life and they just suddenly become enraged. I've seen that happen before, whereas with cannabis usually people just chill out.

Open the Floodgates

Prior to the twentieth century, there was little to no regulation of alcohol and other substances in the United States. Both alcohol and drugs are now subject to strict laws governing their use, possession, and distribution. Starting in the 1970s, with Richard Nixon and passage of the Controlled Substance Act, state and federal lawmakers moved toward what could be considered a zero-tolerance policy regarding illegal drugs, that is, "The War on Drugs."[24] Today, penalties for breaking drug laws are severe and violators often receive long prison sentences for possessing even small amounts of drugs. However, such policies have come under increasing scrutiny. First, there has been a growing awareness and intolerance of the mass incarceration of people of color, especially non-violent drug offenders, who are more heavily policed, charged with drug offenses, and are given longer sentences than are whites. Second, growth in deaths and overdoses due to opioids across demographics (to include middle-class white people) has shifted Americans' attitudes toward drugs from a crime to a public health issue.

The majority of participants felt marijuana should be legalized and regulated and that the financial and medicinal benefits outweigh health and safety concerns. Jan explained, "I actually think about the legalization of marijuana a lot because I do drink alcohol, but I've never done marijuana or drugs of any kind. Like, what's the difference?" And Lori: "In general I'm pretty much like, legalize it and tax the heck out of it. I mean marijuana feels less risky. Obviously still you still shouldn't drive. You're still probably not going to end up in the hospital." Participants told stories of how it's helped with their own health conditions or those of people they know. Nadine said, "I personally don't have a lot of issues with marijuana being legalized. I think about it a little bit differently too, because my cousin's daughter has epilepsy, so she, like, uses CBD oil and stuff like that. There's things like that that have really helped her." Jennifer struggles with chronic pain stemming from her neck and back. She said, "My whole body hurts. It sucks. I have chronic pain. Given my family's history, I was very late to try it. But this winter was so rough on my body. I just did not handle it. So I ended up asking someone, can I try that?

It got me through the winter and it was great because there's no hangover and I don't have any of those blood sugar issues that I do with drinking." Ginny mentioned psychological benefits such as in the case of people with PTSD:

> GINNY: It totally should be legal. I also think that LSD and mushrooms should be explored more for the fact that they can help people get over some really serious shit.

Megan noted that legalizing marijuana could potentially reduce crime: "I think that it actually is going to decrease crime levels, not to mention raise a ton of money, which could be put back into alcohol prevention, drug prevention, and treatment."

Not that there wasn't ambivalence toward legalization, such as with Vera: "I go back and forth on how I feel, and I just feel like I would rather be able to tax it. I would rather be able to monitor it and then be able to get people help easier than make it illegal and treat it like prohibition that nobody will follow anyway." As to whether marijuana should be legal, Bonnie said, "I don't know. There's kind of a catch-22. I mean, if you're going to use it responsibly, that's one thing. I know that medically I think there's a really, really high need for having it be legalized. For my friend it's a medicinal thing. He just knows that it helps control his pain. But is he a pothead? No." Brenda said, "I'm not in love with the idea, I guess. And it's not because . . . well, maybe it is because I'm a prude, I don't know, but I just don't love the idea only because I see it causing harm for people in ways that they don't maybe recognize right now. Kind of like the vaping." And Leigh: "I'm not keen on doing stuff that is illegal. But then I started, like, learning more about it, and it was like, how could we allow ourselves as a society to ban all these other substances and be using opioids for pain and treatment? When this is showing to be way more effective and less harming?"

Participants had two main worries about marijuana—the negative effects on children's development, and driving a car while under the influence. Ella said, "I get if it's very occasionally and you're going out to have fun and you're safe and you have a driver and all that stuff, but it's disheartening I think that it's become legal everywhere. It kind of freaks me out. Like, how many more people can be driving under the influence and what are they doing about *that*?" Sharon worried about that and children's health and their ability to control their consumption: "I think there's enough evidence that under the age of eighteen it's a really bad idea because of chromosomal issues and attention deficit issues and things like that. If a grownup wants to smoke a joint instead of drinking a beer, fine. But kids could eat the whole candy bar without realizing that they're overdosing. You can overdose on THC." In terms of talking about marijuana to their kids, Glenda takes the same approach that she does with alcohol:

GLENDA: You know, so with cannabis I might be a little bit more reserved with it and I would not smoke in front of my kids, just because of the second-hand smoke and they're not consenting to that. But, like, when they get to an age when they can understand it. Probably sixteen would be my number . . .

SUSAN: If they wanted to smoke or take edibles or something like that what would you say?

GLENDA: I mean, I would rather them do it with me than get it from somebody else.

SUSAN: Kind of like alcohol?

GLENDA: Kind of like alcohol. Yeah. I'd probably let them do it. Supervised though. And they're not eating the whole pan. [laughs]

CONCLUSION

This chapter presented women's recollections of what they were told about alcohol as children, and how they are approaching the topic (or would) with their own children. Although these conversations do not provide definitive evidence that attitudes about alcohol are transmitted across generations, they provide some clues. The findings presented here are consistent with those in chapter 2. Lessons about alcohol remained primarily fear-based. Participants with children did not want to appear hypocritical and downplayed previous periods of heavy drinking or opted not to share them with their children at all. However, participants were not immune to changing attitudes and cultural influences. For example, many participants felt that the way Americans approach alcohol is at best unhelpful, and at worst, dangerous. My interviews also suggest that women are becoming more accepting of substances they deem "natural" and see benefits to replacing alcohol with marijuana for themselves and others. Participants overwhelmingly were accepting of marijuana legalization and its use, and some felt it was a healthier and safer option than drinking alcohol. In chapter 4, I continue to explore participants' perceptions of alcohol in society, with a specific focus on how norms and values about alcohol are communicated to women through television, movies, advertising, and social media as well as in workplaces and social activities. I also examine the extent to which social stigma against women's alcohol use remains.

Chapter Four

Reflecting Pools

SHOPPER 1: Remember, Judy doesn't drink.

SHOPPER 2: Is there something wrong?

—Overheard, wine aisle at Target

Recall from chapter 1 that in Colonial America, alcohol was considered acceptable, healthy, and was widely consumed. That changed in the nineteenth century when many Americans came to see using alcohol as immoral and associated it with numerous social problems, and according to a leading commentator, "almost the sole cause of all suffering, the poverty, and the crime to be found in the country."[1] The use of alcohol declined sharply during this period. Women were leaders in the temperance movement against alcohol, which claimed that "alcohol in any form would lead to habitual drunkenness in *anyone* who drank."[2] This movement resulted in the Eighteenth Amendment passed in 1920, which illegalized the manufacture, transportation, and sale of alcohol. Since Prohibition ended in 1933, alcohol consumption steadily increased among both men and women. Today, the majority of Americans drink. They consume alcohol more frequently and in greater amounts. They are more likely to binge drink and to drink chronically. The gap in alcohol use between women and men is nearly closed. Alcohol has pervaded society to the extent that it has become a common feature of previously alcohol-free activities, such as running a race or going to the movies.

In chapter 2, participants provided their definition of *terms*. In this chapter, participants were asked to provide their *definition of the situation*—their perceptions of norms, customs, and expectations for behavior surrounding drinking.[3] My goal was to understand the degree to which alcohol is normalized in the United States, specifically among women. That is, the extent to which drinking alcohol is considered a natural and normal thing for women to do and not considered out of place or shocking in their everyday lives. This is important to reassess given reversals in public attitudes across history. Alcohol's heavy presence on television, movies, commercials, social media, and imagery on products is a good indication of normalization. Such mechanisms are venues for observational learning, educating viewers as to "socially accepted patterns of drinking and drinking situations, common motivations, or consequences of consumption,"[4] and numerous studies have found that exposure to alcohol-related media and advertising shapes drinking attitudes and behavior.[5] Also in this chapter, I explore the normalization of alcohol in the context of women's social activities and employment (parenting is covered in chapter 5). I examine whether women perceive a double standard regarding alcohol consumption in these realms, and the degree to which traditional stereotypes of female drinkers persist.

MEDIA, MEMES, AND WINE SWAG

Media promoting alcohol consumption has traditionally been targeted toward adolescents and young adults (think movies such as *Animal House, American Pie*, and *Mean Girls*). Nowadays, alcohol is pervasive in content meant for older women, female professionals, and mothers, groups not typically associated with heavy drinking. In popular movies such as *Book Club* and *Wine Country* there are few scenes that *don't* include alcohol. Nadine, in her forties, explained: "I think it's kind of like almost more normal now. Like, I think about the things that I watch and they portray it differently [than they used to]. I'm actually rewatching *Grey's Anatomy* right now. They talk about it. They drink tequila. That's their thing."

In previous chapters, I discussed how views on alcohol are heavily polarized, with drinking presented as either great fun or hopelessly tragic. Television and movies bear this out, drawing upon common stereotypes. Participants occupying different stages of the lifecourse picked up on this. Brenda, in her forties, said, "I watch old movies a lot and regular TV and movies. Usually in those movies or TV shows, the women are drinking and they're sassy, and they're funny. Occasionally of course there's the *not* funny drunk woman . . . but that's usually intended to be a funny persona that they have." Ava, who is twenty-five, agrees: "I think anytime I'm seeing something in a movie, it's normally, like, when someone's gone too far, like drunk, hungover, passed out or something. I don't really think I've seen too much in the middle." Sandra, also in her twenties, says in the media alcohol seems necessary "in order to have a good time." She said, "I feel like in most of the movies the crazy adventure happens after they started drinking or partying." And Lori, in her thirties, said, "I just watched *Wine Country*. It's, like, a friend's fortieth birthday or something and so they're all getting together to celebrate and go to different wineries and, you know, drink too much, and hilarity ensues." Vera, who is twenty-five, is an avid reader:

> VERA: I don't think I've read a lot of books where alcohol was put in a good light. I'll say that. Usually if it was mentioned it was because somebody was having a problem with it. They were drinking in excess or altering their behavior with it. Either people are socially drinking, and they're weird because they're *not* drinking, or they're drinking in *way* excess. Like there doesn't seem to be a spectrum.

Several participants expressed discomfort over this: "From a media standpoint, I think sex is demonized a lot more than alcoholism. Like, *The Hangover* really gets me because that whole movie is like, you took random pills from somebody [and] you had a completely terrible experience. I can watch that movie and I can laugh, but that seems really, really bad." "To me it's like, it's not anything attractive. It's not cute. It's not. It's sad. Like in the eighties. Some of those films that had the frat party stuff, where people were drunk and *Sixteen Candles* when the blonde girl was so drunk. It wasn't funny to me. It was absolutely dangerous." Indeed, examples of situations in which women consume alcohol neither socially nor heavily are few and far between. Zoey brought this up:

> ZOEY: I know from personal knowledge that women drink just as much and just as problematic as men do. It's like, I'm going to curl up with a bottle of wine and watch Netflix. I'm starting to see it in women more in their thirties, forties, fifties, and it's not necessarily in a social setting. It's not like, I'm inviting all my friends over to watch the game and we're gonna drink. It's a lot more isolated drinking that I see, but they're not going to show you a sad old woman in her pajamas curled up watching a rom-com, crying. It doesn't seem like the image you're going for.

Social media, websites, and platforms that allow the creation and sharing of content by users, such as Facebook, Twitter, Instagram, and TikTok, have a particularly powerful influence on our ideas, attitudes, and behavior including alcohol.[6] Memes, captioned photos or images that spread quickly through social media, encapsulate messages about alcohol. For example, a meta-analysis of nineteen studies shows that children's engagement with social media (posting, liking, commenting, and viewing alcohol-related content) is associated with higher self-reported drinking and alcohol-related problems.[7] Social media featuring alcohol is associated with greater alcohol consumption and risky drinking in young adults.[8]

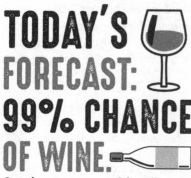

TODAY'S FORECAST: 99% CHANCE OF WINE.

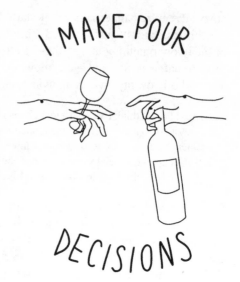

I MAKE POUR DECISIONS

Countless memes on social media make light of women's heavy alcohol use. *Source above*: Ari Sandi/Alamy Stock Vector, Image ID: REH7YW. *Source right*: Pixel Aesthetic/Alamy Stock Vector, Image ID: 2G7CH1P

These platforms tend to be gender-specific and content targeted at women reflects the stresses and strains of *simply being female*. Although midlife and older women are avid users of social media, there has been little research on the effect of alcohol-related social media on their drinking habits. When I asked her about social media, Tracy, a thirty-six-year-old, married project manager, said, "I will tell you, I think [that kind of thing] is hilarious. I saw a meme the other day. This previous week was the first full week of being out of school. It said, 'Can someone help me find the right flavor of wine that goes with my kid being home all day?' Something like that, and I thought it was hilarious." Her husband, whose ex-wife is an alcoholic, was not amused. She continued:

> TRACY: I sent it to my husband, and he responded that it cuts too close to home. Not funny. I thought it was hilarious because my son's autistic and sometimes you want to bang your head against the wall. And I thought he would see that, but he took it very personal. And then we got into it. You know, "you're being insensitive." I was like, okay, I'm done. Let's move on from the conversation.

Alcohol was prevalent in the social media feeds of most participants, typically in carefully curated form. "On Instagram mostly when I'm seeing alcohol it's at the side of a gorgeously plated dish of food." "In terms of social media that I follow, I've got a lot of friends that post glasses of wine. Along with food and stuff like that, and they're saying stuff like, 'relaxing' or 'enjoying a glass of wine.'" "On my Instagram I think a lot of my girlfriends will post if they're going out for dinner and they're getting cocktails or something. It's like that.

It's not usually anybody partying or anything. It's just like, here's my perfect meal and my perfect drink and my perfect life."

Erving Goffman's dramaturgical approach is often applied to understand the role of alcohol in one's presentation of self. A century ago, drinking was viewed as shameful behavior that should be kept "backstage."[9] This remains the case with respect to drinking in excess (aside from binge drinking among college students and young adults). In a study of adolescents with alcoholic parents, the children "loyally performed frontstage appearance as normally as possible."[10] In the technological age, social media is a main venue for impression management and identity construction and "likes" provide instant feedback that helps build one's self-concept. Alcohol is increasingly taking "center stage" with women (and men) performing around it. However, people may have very different ideas as to what is considered appropriate. Ella, who has three kids, was taken aback when she saw others parents posting pictures of themselves drinking on a Facebook page designed to highlight their children's athletic accomplishments.

> ELLA: I don't know how to put it. I feel like I get sucked into teenager peer-pressury feelings because I'll have groups on different social media sites of parents who are part of my children's sporting teams. And many of them will be together and there's always alcohol involved. A lot of alcohol. And what they're posting is "the *fun!*" And so the impression is that you are *boring, not fun*, unless you're posting pictures of you drinking or whatnot.

An overriding theme that emerged from my interviews was that nondrinkers are a drag. A number of participants felt they are receiving more pressure to drink than they had in the past and expressed concern about being labeled "boring." Sandra talks about her college days: "One of my roommates, she felt like she had to drink every Friday night or else it wasn't a weekend. Like, I remember that and how I felt, like, the pressure to drink because she wanted to have a good time. We were really good friends. So, in order to bond with my friends, I had to drink." The pressure to drink has been extended into later adulthood. As Bonnie said, "I would say it's almost like women feel they *have* to. Only because that's what they think they have to do. We're going to go out. We're going to have a girls' night. Let's have wine. I mean, if you want to go to the club and go dancing, you should be able to do it without consuming an obscene amount of alcohol." Diane felt pressure from her sister:

> DIANE: She's a professional. She's successful. We went to Mexico over Christmas together for a girls' trip. And I don't drink very often and, like, my nickname is "two beer Diane" because I have two beers and I, like, giggle and I fall asleep. So my sister is very upset with me that I was not drinking more. She drank as soon as we woke up to as soon as we went to sleep . . . and she'd order

doubles, and she can function! She's like, this is my job. When I go to conferences, I drink. I was like, I do that too but like not like this.

Sociologist Emily Nicolls interviewed twenty-six women between the ages
of eighteen and twenty-five in the "party town" of Newcastle upon Tyne in
northeast England. One participant said women who choose not to drink
were not "not honoring parts of the agreement of going out," highlighting the
"essential nature" of alcohol consumption.[11] Other studies bear this out. An
Australian study of thirty-seven drinking and nondrinking adults by Cheers
and colleagues suggests a growing stigma against nondrinkers.[12] According to
the authors, nondrinkers are a threat to: (a) fun, and cast a judgmental "sober
eye" disruptive to a hedonistic environment, (b) drinkers' ability to make
social connections, and (c) self, in that the presence of nondrinkers cause
drinkers to reflect on their own problematic drinking. Both male and female
drinkers in the study were more accepting of female than male nondrinkers.
Female nondrinkers had an "out," in that they were assumed to be pregnant,
or thinking about getting pregnant, which was considered a legitimate reason
to abstain. Isabel saw this firsthand from people in her martial arts club:

SUSAN: Has anyone ever asked you why you're not drinking?

ISABEL: Yes. We have an alumni event where people from forty years ago all
come back, and if you don't drink at that event, you'll get a lot of questions. I
wasn't drinking because I wanted to be able to go home early. I didn't want to
have to worry about driving. A lot of people asked me if I was pregnant because
I had gotten married and that was the next logical step for them.

SUSAN: And if you said no, what was the reaction?

ISABEL: It depended on the person. The people I know really well would tease
you. If they offered to buy me a drink they'd give me a hard time.

SUSAN: Why do you think they did that?

ISABEL: I think the black belt reunion has, like, a stigma of everybody gets really crazy-drunk. If you're not drinking at a reunion, then it's like what are you
doing there? I get frustrated but I know when they're teasing me. I guess they're
not implying that I'm pregnant. They're just making fun of the fact that I'm not
drinking, which is weird.

Many women noted the increased advertising of alcohol toward women,
playing to common stereotypes, which irritated Olivia and Glenda.

OLIVIA: The marketing has also shifted. You can look at the commercials from
our childhood and other things where it was very targeted towards men. And if

you start looking at it now, it's a social environment. It's a coed, mingled commercial. It's starting to target lighter beverages. Especially in the last couple of years, all of a sudden, we've got the alcoholic seltzer waters and low-calorie alcohol and there's more marketing towards a healthier lifestyle. Let's try to normalize alcohol and make it healthier.

GLENDA: If you look at the grocery store these days and go to the wine aisle, there's a lot of feminine things. It's almost like it's advertised directly for us, it seems like. When they came out with lower calorie wine, it was a big deal. It's like, "Oh, I can have this glass of wine and not bust my caloric intake for the day" or whatever. It was totally geared towards women *achieving*; being able to drink a little bit but within their caloric daily allowance, if you will. I thought it was misogynistic. It's like, I just want regular wine!

In addition to advertising, previously humdrum products, most often kitchen items like coffee mugs and dish towels, have become rife with alcohol-related images and jokes. T-shirts are emblazoned with funny wine-themed sayings and stores are filled with alcohol-related novelty gifts for birthdays and bridal showers. The participants in the study for the most part considered such items harmless fun, like Kim:

KIM: For my wedding night, my bridesmaids surprised me with this *giant* wine glass that holds three bottles of wine. It's like, I'm never gonna drink that myself! [laughs]

SUSAN: Do you still have it?

KIM: No! That thing was taking up way too much space and I don't plan on reusing it! It's like, this is discouraging. You pour a whole bottle in and it's only this far up [uses fingers].

SUSAN: What do you think of those kinds of things?

KIM: It's insane. It's silly. Kind of like a gag gift of sorts is what I think of them. But I can see where people would take them seriously. Or, like the bras where you can put the wine and stuff in them or whatever. Or the purse? They crack me up. But I would *never* personally own one.

Megan has a number of alcohol-related items:

MEGAN: I have a wine glass for sure. I've got a funny dish towel someone gave me. I've definitely gotten, like, birthday cards where it's like, you know, "Like fine wine, we're better when we age," or something stupid like that. I know I'd probably give it to them too. So yeah. It's funny. It's cute. It's light. It doesn't bother me. I mean, I don't take it as anything in particular.

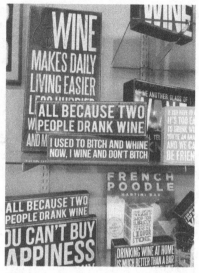 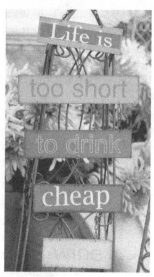

"Wine swag" seems to have taken over the women's gift market. *Source left*: Patti McConville/Stockimo/Alamy Stock Photo, Image ID: S283BY. *Source right*: Tim Gainey/Alamy Stock Photo, Image ID: BP7667

Lotta Dann, creator of the online community Living Sober and author of *The Wine O'Clock Myth*, provides a scathing critique of "women and wine culture." She makes similar observations regarding the infiltration of alcohol in advertising, television, movies, social media, clothing, and household products meant for women. She complains:

> As for greeting cards, don't get me started. Every time I go to choose a birthday, anniversary, or some other type of congratulatory card I end up sifting through a bunch about alcohol: "It's your birthday, time to get wrecked!"; "Let's get into the holiday spirit."; "Dear wine, be my Valentine." Sometimes it's hard to find a card that *isn't* booze-related.[13]

There is even a movement underway called #dontpinkmydrink, which Dann explains, "highlights how alcohol brands are cynically marketing alcohol to women, piggybacking on empowerment movements and natural female camaraderie to sell their products."[14]

DRINK LIKE A GIRL

Despite growth in women's alcohol consumption, the media, advertising, and products typically draw on traditional notions of femininity, suggesting the continuation of a double standard for women. Tracy said, "There's a lot of memes out there. You know, guys waking up next to the big girl or the ugly girl, you know, the caption says something like, 'Um, gee, never going to do another Jäger bomb again!' You know, it's always a slight against a woman."

> BRENDA: You go to a kitchen store and there's *always* a fifties mom sort of "prim and proper, but I'm a little bit naughty . . ." Lots of stuff like that. A lot of the wines and alcohols, but wines specifically, are marketed, it seems like, specifically towards women. Like the Cupcake wine and the Skinny Girl wine. I mean, I can't imagine my dad pulling out a bottle of Cupcake!

According to historian Rocco Capraro, alcohol consumption has always been a "male domain." Drinking alcohol falls into "a line of masculine icons, including body building, sexual assault, and pornography."[15] Male drinking is associated with stereotypical, generally positive, male traits such as acting as a leader and a willingness to take risks.[16] Women who drink experience significantly greater societal disapproval than do men and are considered less feminine and more sexually available than woman who do not imbibe.[17] In an experiment, women shown in a social setting with a beer, as opposed to water, were "dehumanized" (deemed lacking in human qualities such as morality, self-restraint, and warmth) to a greater degree by men *and women*, especially if they appeared intoxicated. There was no corresponding effect when men were shown.[18] In the study of Australian drinkers mentioned previously, one participant put it this way: "Drunken men are seen to be dangerous and drunken women are seen to be vulnerable. I think that there's this very clear binary in how a man drunk and walking off from a party makes people nervous and a woman walking off drunk from a party makes people nervous, but for different reasons."[19]

To explore the existence of a double standard, I asked participants to respond to two basic fill-in-the-blank questions. First, "Men who drink are . . ." About a third of participants provided answers along the lines of "normal," "fine," and "typical" or used phrases such as "whatever they want to be." Another third or so of participants had trouble articulating a response: "Nothing's really coming into my head," "I don't have anything . . . there's nothing there," "Oh gosh, umm, it shouldn't be this hard," and "my mind totally went blank." The question prompted Melanie to reflect on her family: "I don't visit terribly often, but, like, as a typical day for my dad, like on a Saturday morning, he'll go to the store and he'll come back with a six pack of tall beers and he'll just sit the whole day and drink. Then I have several male relatives who just drink a lot all the time with no purpose but just to drink. Not socially, it's just ingrained in their everyday life."

I posed the same question in reference to women (i.e., "Women who drink are . . . "). Here, participants' answers were more nuanced. Although a few participants responded "normal" or "fine," the most common responses by far were along the lines of "fun," "lighthearted," and "chatty." Two women said "stressed," and another said, "drinking alone." One said, "unhappy," and one said, "judged." Christine said, "I think for many women there's sort of like a question mark above our heads when it comes to this." Overall, participants' responses are consistent with stereotypes of women drinkers as either fun party girls or sad basket cases. Participants provided more details and context when they talked about women who drink than they did when talking about men. "I guess when I think of women and drinking I think mostly of fun or celebratory types of things, like going out for a drink to celebrate x, y, z, or I'm having my friends over." "I immediately think, like, going to the wine bar and having, like, a chilled glass of wine and, like, talking about your problems or something." "I see it manifesting in different ways. In men, I think of fragile masculinity and this bravado, and for women I think of nights of hysteria and crying and things like that." "From what I hear and see on social media, it's just like, 'I'm so stressed out. I can't wait to go home and have a drink' or whatever. Sometimes one of my friends even jokes, 'Alcohol's cheaper than therapy.'" This led me to the conclusion that women's use of alcohol seemed to require a *reason*, such as to celebrate with friends or cope with stress, whereas men's use of alcohol did not.

Furthermore, women's drinking was more often seen as a symptom of underlying issues—either childhood neglect or trauma, overwhelming stressors, or loneliness, whereas men who drink *just drink*. The HBO series *The Flight Attendant* portrays an attractive young woman in a glamorous profession, jet-setting around the world visiting exotic locales and partying with friends. It is soon apparent that this same woman is heavily alcohol dependent (she carries a flask and drinks vodka all day, even on the job), is an unreliable friend, coworker, and family member, is sexually promiscuous, and blacks out not infrequently. As is so often the case in movies and television, her drinking is connected to a major trauma from her past. Her drinking has dire consequences when she wakes up and her one-night stand is dead and she has no idea what happened. There is an overtone of lack of personal responsibility and victim blaming and "you reap what you sow." Television and movies also perpetuate the notion that women who drink inevitably fall victim to sexual assault. *Law and Order SVU* was mentioned by participants more than once, as Megan stated, "I was just watching *Law and Order*. The guy was slipping her a mickey. I don't know what they call them? In her drink, you know, and then raping the girls, a not great TV show."

According to Bonnie, "When women get together and go out, it's kind of that double-edged sword and that catch-22 again because guys can drink, but women shouldn't." A number of participants worried about how their drinking would be perceived by others:

PARKER: I think women and alcohol, generally speaking, is a little more subdued in relation to men. Like a little more responsible. Like, what if they think I'm a big lush? Because I say that I get drunk sometimes, so there was kind of like a concern that I would be misrepresented by somebody else because I drank at all.

SUSAN: Do you think if you were a man you would feel the same way?

PARKER: I don't know. Maybe not. I think that men get more of a pass about drinking alcohol. I feel like I have to be very responsible about it. I think there's a difference. I don't think there should be a difference, but I think there is a difference.

Although alcohol consumption by women is often seen as an indicator of gender equality, Christine's remarks also suggest the continuance of a double standard.

CHRISTINE: Maybe the one place where we reached equality is that some of expectations of being a demure, always sober woman have been lifted? I mean I guess I don't notice it in . . . necessarily . . . wait, that's not true! I volunteer at the school a lot and sometimes some of the mothers there will mention how much they're looking forward to going home and having a beer, or a glass of wine. No one says, "I'm looking forward to going home and drinking a six pack." But it is sort of more of an undercurrent. Why? It was always acceptable for men to, for dads, or for men to be drinking even to excess.

Overall, participants perceived a greater expectation of responsibility and control for female drinkers. As Isabel explained, "I think there's just a certain level of, like, shame, I guess, of women going out and binge drinking, especially if they're getting dressed up, like when you drive downtown on a Friday night. You don't notice the drunk men as much as you notice the drunk girls." Emily Nicholls, in her study of young female drinkers in England, sought to understand how women navigate the "night time economy" in a supposedly post-feminist world. She found that women must work hard to drink "strategically" to achieve what criminologist Fiona Measham refers to as a "controlled loss of control."[20] As one of Nicholls's participants said, "It's pretty difficult because you basically have to try and get rid of all your inhibitions while not getting rid of everything else . . . And it's quite tricky, I generally fail at it."[21]

GIRL POWER

Throughout the world, women drink less alcohol than do men on every measure of alcohol consumption.[22] The size of the disparity varies across cultures and historical eras. Because alcohol falls within the male domain, differences in alcohol consumption (amount, type, location) are indicators of male privilege and provide information on gender roles and the status of women. In societies where the status of women is low (where they have less education and less access to paid employment), men drink substantially more than women. In cultures with more equity between men and women, the gender disparity is much smaller. For example, American Indian women have a relatively high level of authority in their communities historically and today.[23] The gender gap in alcohol consumption, binge drinking, and AUDs is substantially smaller among American Indians than Blacks, Asians, and Hispanics.[24] Women in Brazil have been gaining ground with substantial growth in female labor force participation, wages, and education, and a 2005 study found no disparity in baseline abstinence between Brazilian women and men.[25] One of my participants, Leigh, is from Brazil:

> LEIGH: And what I notice is that I didn't think as much about my gender when I lived there as I do here. I never thought that my gender was limiting towards what I could accomplish career-wise. Like women were doing better in college than men. Within my family, even though the two people I can think of that had an alcohol problem were men, it wasn't that men drink and women didn't, right? Everybody drank.

According to Nicholls, "Women are told they can finally 'have it all' and are compelled to be confident, assertive, and pleasure-seeking and to strive for success in an individualized and competitive—rather than collective—way in all spheres of their lives."[26] This trend is not necessarily well received. One way that opposition to women's independence has manifested itself is through what Nicholls refers to as the "girling" of women, which diminishes any gains in power by continued expectations of traditional feminine beliefs, practices, and behavior, such as caring about clothes and wearing makeup. For example, the "Girl Power" movement of the 1990s was a form of "active girlhood" based on assertiveness and individual achievement while valuing traditional femininity focusing on friendships, fun, and sassiness.[27] Promoting "girlness" is certainly admirable but has also opened women and girls up to mockery and trivialization, and whether girls have benefited from this movement is the subject of debate.[28] Girling can be seen as part of what gender scholars Lisa Wade and Myra Marx Feree refer to as *the feminine apologetic* or "how a woman's performance of femininity can be a way to soothe others' concerns about her appropriation of masculinity."[29]

Women's steady movement into formerly male drinking spaces challenges dominant attitudes that only men drank in public. The solution? Girling. In "How Babycham Changed British Drinking Habits," Ben Milne describes how Babycham (a sparkling "perry" or pear cider) became the first alcoholic beverage marketed to women, with Babycham providing "a glimpse of a new, more glamorous and aspirational world arising from the ashes of post-WW2 austerity and rationing." According to historian Pete Brown, cited in the article, "Babycham was posh, it was sophisticated, it was advertised on the telly. It became a symbol."[30] Philip Norman, author of *Babycham Night*, said, "Babycham was the first drink a woman could order in a bar without feeling like a tart or a crone."[31] Although Babycham disappeared in the 1970s, "drinks for women" continue to evolve in the form of wines, mixed drinks, and spiked seltzers, with "babychams" making a comeback in the form of handcrafted hard ciders and juice-infused beer.

To further gauge the double standard, I asked participants directly, "What comes to mind when thinking about women and alcohol?" Their responses suggest that women have internalized these types of gendered messages about what women should be drinking and under what conditions. Participants typically spoke of girls' night and wine bars. Joellyn said, "I do automatically think wine." Tabitha said, "I just immediately think more wine versus if I'm thinking of a man, my immediate thought is, like, beer," and Diane: "When you think of women you think of fruity, girly drinks versus the stereotype for men, who drink beer and whiskey. Things like that." Not to say that there weren't women who rebelled against girling, such as Kim, who said, "I mean, females are just more associated with wine coolers and the fruity stuff. Because we're *notorious* for having the fruity stuff which was why I was like, no, I'm not gonna be that person. I'm drinking a Guinness."

OUTLAW WOMEN

Kim was not alone. A number of participants were annoyed, if not fed up, with stereotypes of women drinkers. Janet and Ginny are in their twenties. They both brought up a television show based on a Marvel comic book character who makes no apologies for heavy drinking:

JANET: I *love* Jessica Jones! She's a great example of a straight-up alcoholic. Her superpower is that she can lift super heavy things, she can, like, crush things. She's like grungy, dungy, fuck the world, I hate everything. I'm going to sit down here with a bottle of Jack. It's not really seen as a positive thing. It's seen as her way of dealing with her past trauma. Her character goes through gaslighting and rape and her whole family died in an accident. There's this whole series of tragedies.

SUSAN: What do you think that says about society that that's really popular?

JANET: I see it as this is a really positive thing. There are women out there. There are women who are angry. There are women who are drunks. There are women who are abusive. There are women who are terrible people. And, like, we never see women who are terrible people. Like, we're just goddesses. We're just ready to have babies. But there's other kinds of women. To me that's nice, because I like to see both sides.

GINNY: They definitely show her looking like pretty rough. She does a lot of dangerous behavior like random sex with people and getting wasted and, like, not being a very good friend. It's kind of nice to have a show where it's kind of like, oh, hey, here's somebody who's dealing with some shit and they're definitely not doing it in a healthy way, but it's not just like this, oh, everything has to be all happy and sunshine! [in sing-song voice].

In *Wine Country*, the wine flows and acts as a kind of truth serum. Tina Fey plays Tammy, the rough-around-the-edges Airbnb owner who tells it like it is. She advises the women, "The Wi-Fi here is very slow, so you're just going to have to talk to each other . . . while drinking a ton of wine! What could possibly go wrong? Just remember, guys, whatever gets said, is probably what the person has always felt, and the alcohol just lets it out."

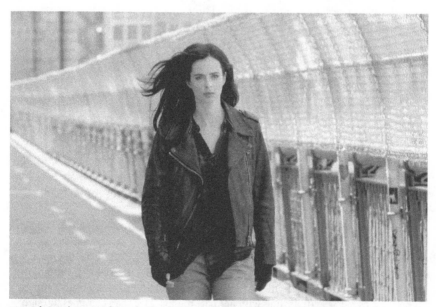

Marvel Comics superhero Jessica Jones drinks unapologetically. *Source*: Atlaspix/Alamy Stock Photo, Image #FBPBWT

WOMEN'S WORK

Over the past century, especially the last fifty years, women have steadily moved into the paid workforce and occupations and work roles previously considered "males only." This trend is an important one in relation to alcohol consumption. In the U.S. and globally, women who are more educated and employed, especially college graduates in professional occupations, are more likely to drink and use alcohol in higher amounts.[32] Many of my participants linked increased drinking among women to women's empowerment and their greater representation in the media, politics, social life, and especially with respect to work, like Olivia:

> OLIVIA: Drinking just wasn't visible because women were more seen and not heard. I think it has more to do with how society has changed and women have shown that we can do just about anything: study, work, balance, and really starting to normalize that balance and relationships. Plus I've watched marketing change. We used to have Joe Camel and the Marlboro Man and you had the Virginia Slims commercials for the women. Or the Enjoli [perfume] commercials, you know, "I can bring home the bacon, fry it up in a pan."

The mid-nineteenth century might be considered the heyday of alcohol and work culture, at least among white men in the professional class (think *Mad Men* and the three-martini lunch). With the onset of the recession of the 1970s, drinking alcohol at work came to be seen as wasteful and self-indulgent, and female employees argued that business being conducted after hours at happy hour and golf courses left women out of networking and mentoring opportunities. Even so, in a 2018 study of TV workplace dramas (e.g., *The Good Wife*, *House of Cards*, *The Newsroom*), 90 percent of episodes contained representations or references to alcohol, and nearly one-third of all beverages consumed at work were alcoholic. Moreover, few negative consequences of alcohol consumption were shown.[33] In reality, a nationally representative survey of nearly three thousand employed adults indicated that "workplace alcohol use and impairment" directly affected an estimated 15 percent of the U.S. workforce, either through alcohol use at work, working under the influence of alcohol, or working with a hangover, and 7 percent, or nine million workers, reported drinking during their workday.[34] The costs of alcohol consumption to employees and employers in the form of accidents and fatalities, reduced productivity, and absenteeism are rarely discussed.[35]

Drinking *after* work, however, has been shown to have positive outcomes for individuals and the workplace environment. Based on interviews with twenty-six Norwegian managers and employees across several business sectors, it was concluded that drinking after work created collective experiences, strengthened bonds between colleagues, and provided a "transition ritual" between work and home. Several managers in that study encouraged their employees to drink together. One said, "It's about building relationships and getting to know each other informally. You want to have a good team that works well together," and another said, "It's a good thing that they head out and get really drunk afterwards. Because you have a level of stress and such an extreme pressure at work that you need to get it out of your system."[36]

As noted in chapter 1, numerous studies show a link between work stress and alcohol consumption. In a nationally representative survey of U.S. workers, work-related stressors (e.g., too little time to complete tasks) were found to increase one's risk of experiencing unpleasant emotions such as depression, anxiety, and hostility, which in turn were associated with elevated alcohol use.[37] Relieving stress was a common reason my participants said they drank after work with colleagues. Ava used to work at a big box store. She and her coworkers often got together after work. She said, "It was a very stressful job. We're just cashiering, so you wouldn't think that'd be bad, but there was never anyone scheduled. And the only thing that got you through the day was like, okay, we're going to get drinks after work. Like, I can make it through this. You just use it to kind of cope with the stress and the 'fun' of [the store], if you will."

Many high-status and high-pressure occupations traditionally occupied by men are associated with heavy alcohol use, such as sales, medicine, academia, and law. As Devon Jersild writes in *Happy Hours: Alcohol in a Woman's Life*, among attorneys, there is substantial pressure to socialize formally and informally with clients and colleagues where alcohol is almost always present, at restaurants and country clubs, parties, and weekend retreats.[38] Failing to do so "can knock you off a partnership track, for in these social contexts, lawyers make connections, showcase their strengths, and are informally evaluated by their colleagues." She argues that women either join in or get left out. The use of alcohol in work settings has been increasingly normalized across occupations and employment sectors. For example, many participants had received alcohol-related items from coworkers. As Brenda told me: "Just this year, I got some things for a project that I finished that was big. A friend at work gave me a little bottle of champagne and one of those insulated stemless wine cups as a gift, which was really sweet. I've used it more for juice than wine!" Alcohol was an integral part of the workplace culture for some participants. Bonnie talks about her first job after graduation. She said,

BONNIE: It was awful because the owner of the business had such a mindset to go out and party after our shifts. There was a bar across the street, and it was kind of piggybacked by a restaurant. So we'd go out to eat and then go party it up until closing.

SUSAN: Like you felt like that was an extension of your job and you had to go?

BONNIE: It was kind of expected that you go socially. I think I might have been one of the only ones that was married, and it's like, I don't want to do this. I want to go home and spend time with my husband. But yeah, it was very much a part of it.

In some occupations, such as sales, it is common to drink in the context of work.

DIANE: We go to a lot of conferences. I go to a conference, find some people, take them out to dinner, and go to the bars. They go really hard and they'll be out till three o'clock in the morning and they are plastered drunk. And you've just met them. You have to get them home, make sure that they're safe. And since I started school [in that industry], I've noticed a really similar trend among my classmates that when they have a chance to drink, they drink *a lot*. And it's usually a very long night.

Parker talked about her time as a teacher in South Korea.

PARKER: They have a lot of pressure on them at home and at work, but they also have a lot of social freedom to get drunk, release that stress, and then go back to work.

SUSAN: Is that for women too?

PARKER: Yeah. I mean, it's more for men, but women too. I worked in an elementary school that was almost all women. We would go for teacher dinners once every few months and everyone was expected to get drunk.

The availability of alcohol at the workplace, perceptions of the acceptability of drinking at work, and the drinking of coworkers are, not surprisingly, strong predictors of work-related drinking.[39] Along with other amenities, alcohol is relatively common at start-ups and tech companies that want to appear "hip" and "cool," and is often used as a recruiting tool to attract the best and brightest employees. However, alcohol in a work environment was not necessarily welcomed among participants. This was the case for Ginny, who works at a tech company that focuses on financial services:

GINNY: We have a beer fridge at my work, and on Fridays I have to go and figure out which beer I'm gonna drink because I'm like, which one can I drink in two hours and won't get drunk? That's, like, a decision I have to make. Because I don't drink that often or that much.

SUSAN: Why is there a beer fridge at your work?

GINNY: There is a beer fridge that opens every Friday at three p.m. and there's also wine. So you can have beer or wine. There's also nonalcoholic things in there. There's like La Croix and soda so it's just kind of like a part of the culture.

SUSAN: Can you drink as much as you want? How does that work?

GINNY: I think it's just like, it exudes this certain . . . like when your company does that I think it just kind of makes everybody realize how relaxed an environment it is and it just is very, like, trusting? And so I think they open the beer fridge for things like that and use it for a motivator because a lot of people are like, yeah, it is super-cool that I can have a beer at work.

Several participants agreed that having alcohol available at the office could be difficult to navigate. Ginny noted: "I think because you're allowed to drink at work it automatically makes everybody a little scared to drink at work. Because like, oh, God, I don't want to be the person who gets wasted at work and makes an ass out of myself in front of my boss." Then, too, social media also makes it possible for employers to scrutinize their employees' drinking behavior.

PARKER: I think that even when maybe someone's like, "Yeah, I drink," and they're happy to say that in certain company, you know, close friends, they maybe don't want their boss to know that they drink as much as they do, or they don't want, you know, pictures of themselves drinking on social media because they know that there's this question mark of like, what does that . . . what kind of person does that make me look like?

Glenda works at a daycare center.

GLENDA: The people I work with are probably a good eight years younger than me, so they're definitely going out to the bars and, you know, having those drinks with friends or whatever. They'll tag each other on Facebook and check in, but you don't actually know how much they're consuming because it's just, "Here with the girls," and they'll tag each other but they don't say, "Well we just had twelve pints," because you know we have a lot of parents on Facebook, so we try to kind of dial that down a bit, but yeah, at work I see the drinking culture a lot more than in my personal social circle.

Some participants mentioned it being potentially awkward for colleagues who don't drink:

CARLY: It's a smaller company. Like, if we have a great day—a good record month or whatever—we'll go out and get some drinks on the company. We had a bags tournament during work hours. Our boss bought us beer . . . it's part of the culture there.

SUSAN: Why do you think they do that?

CARLY: I think it's because we're just a small company. We're like a family and we all, well, most of us drink and so we just go out and celebrate, typically.

We have one person who's a recovering alcoholic and we respect that. She still attends. Our Christmas white elephant gifts do include alcohol, which I sometimes feel a little uncomfortable about just because for a recovering alcoholic, you know, that's tough.

CONCLUSION

In this chapter I explored the extent to which alcohol has become normalized for women. I gathered information on women's perceptions of alcohol in conventional media (television, movies, advertising), social media, social activities, and the workplace as potential mechanisms for normalization. Whether or not the presence of alcohol in these environments is capable of changing women's attitudes toward drinking (and drinking behavior) is a question that cannot be answered as a result of these conversations. However, prior research indicates that these forces can have powerful effects on peoples' attitudes and behavior including alcohol consumption.

My interviews are consistent with other studies pointing to increased normalization of alcohol consumption, and that expectation extends to women. Regardless of the level of alcohol they themselves consumed, participants provided many examples of how alcohol is firmly embedded in their everyday lives and surroundings. As was the case for *people who drink*, most participants had absorbed mainstream perceptions of *women who drink*. Their social media presented alcohol as elegant, sophisticated, and fun or as a harmless solution to women's very real frustration with children, partners, and jobs. Similar to alcohol consumption more broadly, entertainment presents women's drinking in a polarized way: moderate, occasional drinking with a husband or group of girlfriends on the one hand, and alcoholism, isolation, and victimization on the other. Alcohol appears to be increasingly expected at women's workplaces and social settings, even those involving children.

Whereas some participants were not overly concerned with this, others felt uneasy about what these messages are communicating to women about femininity, social roles, and their value in society. Whereas a double standard of drinking appears to have lessened for women, it definitely persists. Women must walk a fine line in terms of the amount they drink, the type of alcohol they consume, where they consume it, and with whom. Women who drink must be careful. Women who drink must be in control. Women who drink should be feminine but not too girly. Women who drink must do so for a reason. That is, unlike men, women are still not allowed to enjoy alcohol *for its own sake*. Chapter 5 examines these issues specifically in relation to mothers, for whom drinking is even more treacherous.

Chapter Five

Treading Water

SUSAN: What is happening that women are drinking more?

JENNIFER: What do I think is going on? I think they're stressed out. Women have started to join the workforce, but men have not started to share the households and the emotional work of the family. Women are still doing almost a hundred percent of the housework. They're still doing a hundred percent of the cooking and grocery shopping. They're still signing the kids up for soccer and basketball and driving them places. And dads just show up. I would say in the vast majority of my beautiful, suburban, upscale, middle-class neighborhood, the dad does jack shit. He goes to work and comes home and that's enough. And the mom does everything and also works full time. So the moms feel overwhelmed and they feel like they're losing the battle no matter what they do.

—Jennifer, age 43, married, two children

Women's alcohol consumption tends to decline with age, but it is not necessarily a steady progression. Drinking is sensitive to major life events, increasing and/or plateauing with some transitions (going to college, divorce, the empty nest) and decreasing with others (employment, marriage, and motherhood).[1] However, anecdotal evidence (e.g., articles on social media, memes, blog posts) suggests that mothers are drinking more than in times past. At the time of this writing, empirical studies tracking alcohol consumption among women with children are scarce (an important question for demographers going forward). An exception is a study by epidemiologists Sarah McKetta and Katherine Keyes, who examined the drinking patterns of women who were part of the National Health Interview Study.[2] They found that women with children were more likely to abstain from alcohol and were less likely to binge drink or drink heavily than women without children. However, their

73

analysis also showed that binge drinking and heavy drinking have increased among mothers and non-mothers alike, while abstinence declined.

Other evidence indirectly suggests that drinking has increased among mothers. Alcohol consumption, binge drinking, and alcohol-related liver disease have risen most among women in midlife, the majority of whom have children.[3] Several studies suggest an uptick in mothers' alcohol consumption when their adult children "leave the nest."[4] And the same forces that transformed women's roles also transformed those held by mothers. Women with children are increasingly college educated, employed, and have higher earnings than in the past, statuses associated with higher rates of alcohol consumption.[5] The educational, employment, and income gap between women with children and without children has shrunken considerably.[6]

Although mothers' work lives have transformed, their home lives have not. They are still responsible for the bulk of childcare and housework. Women do nearly twice as much housework as men and spend significantly more time on daily "core" housework (cooking, cleaning, laundry, etc.).[7] And although fathers' involvement with their children has increased over the decades, mothers still do nearly twice the amount of childcare than do fathers and spend more time on routine care, such as feeding and bathing.[8] Even working mothers do the majority of housework and childcare, putting in an unpaid "second shift" of labor on top of paid employment. In families with children under age eighteen, 80 percent of women say they are usually the one to prep and cook meals and 80 percent say they are responsible for the grocery shopping. Mothers also have substantial "kin keeping" responsibilities—remembering birthdays, planning and executing holiday celebrations, making doctor's appointments, organizing children's activities and playdates, volunteering for school events, and so on.[9] Mothers, especially married mothers, have less leisure time than men for socializing, exercise, and personal activities than do fathers, and get less sleep.[10] On top of that, mothers' leisure time is "contaminated" by multitasking childcare and other domestic labor, and they experience more fragmentation and interruptions in leisure.[11]

Then, too, single mothers account for one-quarter of all families with children under age eighteen, and are generally solely responsible for their children's care.[12] It is not news that these families are financially stretched. Only one-half of custodial mothers have child support orders, and less than half (46 percent) who are supposed to receive child support received their full payments.[13] Single mothers are more socially isolated than are partnered mothers and feel less supported by the people in their lives. Never-married and divorced mothers spend more time than married mothers alone and engaging in passive leisure activities (mostly watching television). Single women have fewer social ties and stress-buffering resources, experience greater stress, and are in worse psychological and physical health, all of which are associated with greater alcohol consumption.[14]

In this chapter, I provide participants' impressions of mothers who use alcohol and the reasons they attribute to their drinking. Specifically, I was interested in exploring the idea that mothers drink alcohol to cope with relentless work and family demands. Studies have found the strain between work and family roles negatively affects women's physical and psychological health and is associated with the use of alcohol and other drugs.[15] Results from a 1995 survey indicated that "spillover" of work pressures to family life (e.g., stress makes you irritable at home, job worries or problems distract you when you are at home) was associated with alcohol problems.[16] Similarly, a 1993 study of adults residing in Erie County, New York, showed interference of work with family life is associated with higher rates of heavy alcohol consumption among women.[17] In a nationally representative telephone survey conducted between 2008 and 2011, women who believed alcohol helps reduce tension, and who are experiencing greater work stress, are more likely to drink heavily.[18] These studies are suggestive of a link, but they are quantitative in nature, were conducted over a decade ago, or were based on nonrepresentative samples. There are few studies containing the personal narratives of stress, motherhood, and alcohol use.

In a 2017 national survey, 77 percent of women said they felt a lot of pressure to be an involved parent compared to 49 percent of men, and 60 percent of mothers reported it is very or somewhat difficult to balance the responsibilities of work and family compared to 52 percent of men.[19] In another, 37 percent of mothers said they are "always rushed" compared to 29 percent of fathers.[20] In study of one hundred mothers who completed residential treatment for addiction, the most common reason they listed for drinking was "stress and anxiety related to motherhood."[21] Women who subscribe to traditional gender expectations for women are at greater risk of substance use.[22]

MOTHERS' LITTLE HELPER

Mothers have always been held responsible for their children's successes and failures and have been blamed for everything from schizophrenia to autism. The individualistic and competitive culture of the United States, combined with poor institutional supports for families (e.g., reliable childcare, flexible schedules, paid family leave), compounds the pressures on mothers. Moreover, the bar has been raised as to what constitutes a "good" parent. Sociologist Sharon Hayes put a name to this phenomenon, *intensive mothering*. Intensive mothering involves the close supervision of children, high levels of involvement in children's academics and activities, continuous monitoring of children's achievement, and self-sacrifice, putting others' needs above one's own.[23] This parenting style has become the desired model of raising children, if not standard. In her article "How Mommy Drinking Culture Has Normalized Alcoholism for Women in America," Sarah Cottrell states, "Wine has practically become the must-have accessory for modern motherhood," calling the day-to-day demands placed on mothers "dizzying and never-ending."[24] It's probably no accident that the rise in women's alcohol use coincided with this trend. Mothers may be using drinking as a way to cope with the anxiety of "doing it wrong" and daily stressors and, according to Pamela Raine, just to "get by."[25] From this perspective, drinking is not self-indulgent nor selfish. Drinking allows women, especially mothers, to function in the face of overwhelming demands. Tracy is married and has one child of her own and two stepchildren:

> TRACY: All I can think is, like, give me my iPad and don't speak to me for an hour. I just need to decompress. So those are usually moments where I'm like, "Oh, I'll just pour glass of wine." And I have a really bad habit of not being able to sit down in my own home. I'm always running around dusting and organizing. And so here I am carrying my glass of wine, you know, around the kitchen and vacuuming. And so I always seem to have this glass of wine with me. And I don't know if it's the guilt of I'm not spending time with my son, or just boredom. So I struggled with that. I'm like, "Well, is it okay that I'm drinking half a bottle of wine before dinner?" Because I've diluted it with three cans of sparkling water and a ton of ice. It's almost like I try to rationalize and compromise in my own brain.

Decades ago, a "little yellow pill" was prescribed to millions of disenchanted, anxious, and mildly (or profoundly) depressed women in the 1960s, women who should "have it all"—marriage, children, and a lovely home in the suburbs. As Betty Friedan writes in the preface of the tenth anniversary edition of her 1963 book *The Feminine Mystique*, "I, like other women, thought there was something wrong with *me* because I didn't have an orgasm waxing the kitchen floor."[26] All that's changed is that mother's little helper comes in the form of a glass of chardonnay:

> SHARON: I've noticed this particularly on social media in the last five years—a lot of mommy drinking, that it's become, and I don't know where all of this started, but it's become okay to talk about, you know, coping. I mean, it used to be the Valium. When I was kid, it was the Valium mom.
>
> SUSAN: Mother's little helper, right?
>
> SHARON: Mother's little helper, yeah. And maybe people are just not hiding it the same way they used to. But yeah, there's a lot of mommy drinking, which

bothers me. Because I don't think it's good for little kids to see their mothers drunk. I don't like seeing people get hurt. It's sad to think that people's home lives are so difficult that a bottle of vodka is necessary at the end of the week.

In "Scary Mommy Confessions: When You're a Mom Who Drinks," a stay-at-home mom writes, "At three o'clock, after a long day of rule policing and laundry folding, I feel its familiar pull. As the day begins to fade and beams of late evening sun filter through my kitchen windows, I start to feel antsy. *No, I tell myself. Not yet. It's too early. You should wait.*"[27] My participants were not unaware of what appears to be mothers' increased reliance on alcohol. They were overwhelmingly sympathetic, whether or not they were mothers themselves.

> LEIGH: I was watching a show the other day and this woman is home with her kids and she's, like, drinking wine. And her husband comes in unexpectedly during lunchtime and she tries to hide the alcohol. And I'm like, my grandfather never did that, you know? And he was an alcoholic and he actually had an issue. So I think there's still a lot of shame. Maybe that's why we have so many memes, because people want assurance that what they're doing is okay.

> SELA: When I see memes, at first it's like, oh, that's funny. And then it goes to that deeper level where I'm just like, that's not funny because there's a struggling mom who actually needs help. What are we doing to tell her it's okay to get help? Maybe that's what we're missing. As more women have those competing pressures, what are we going to say? You feel sad. You feel depressed, postpartum, whatever it is that you're feeling anxiety and pressure about; don't just have another glass of wine. Like, what can you do to figure out some tools to help you?

Mothers drink for reasons other than to relieve stress. Women's lives change dramatically with the introduction of children. Anthropologist Ben Killingsworth conducted an ethnographic study of middle-class mothers from Melbourne, Australia, who participated in a playgroup with other mothers of young children. His findings suggest that alcohol was important in maintaining their previous identities as childless women and the independence afforded to women without children. The women told many stories of their lives before becoming mothers, such as going out to pubs with their friends. Telling anecdotes from their past lives allowed them to "draw on that power." One participant remarked rather optimistically that when their children are old enough to be in school they could drink champagne cocktails all afternoon. Others joked about drinking the cooking wine while preparing dinner because it needed "plenty of testing." Alcohol provided these mothers with reassurance, if only among themselves, that they were more than just "stay-at-home mums."[28]

Motherhood is stressful though. Sela is married and has children of her own. She is also raising the children of her sister, who passed away as a result of chronic alcohol abuse. She explains, "It's like we kind of made it okay. You know, the whole kind of 'misery loves company.' Like, I'm breaking. You're breaking. Let's all just let our kids play and have a glass of wine [laughter]. Now you can text a picture of your wine to your mommy friend and be like, 'I'm done for the night. How about you?'"

> JENNIFER: The girls in the neighborhood started a book club, which is more of a wine club than a book club, really. Let's see . . . What else did we do? Oh, we do Girls' Club. Once a month hang out. We don't technically do it anymore, but there's still a core little group of girls that want to go have dinner, go to a concert or whatever, but we almost always get stupid drunk.

Low-income women, especially single mothers, generally have less time and money for this kind of thing, and as noted previously drink less alcohol than do middle-class women. Zoey had been a single mother but is in a professional occupation (a therapist). She describes drinking heavily after her separation and a new shared custody arrangement with her soon to be ex-husband.

> ZOEY: The nights the kids would be with him, I would drink most nights. Because I just hated not being with my family that wasn't there anymore. So it was a coping thing. I would sit at home by myself and I would drink. It was beer. Sometimes it could be six, seven, eight, nine beers?
>
> SUSAN: Over the course of the evening?
>
> ZOEY: Yes. Like from the time I got home from work until I went to bed. So that started, and then I got an OWI. I had gone to an anniversary party. It was at a Mexican restaurant, and I had margaritas, and then I got ready to leave the restaurant, and I did kind of a turn where it wasn't exactly like I should have, and there was a policeman there and he saw me and I blew over. So then I was scared. I was like, "Oh my God, what have I done?" My career? Like, I was back to working by that time, and I was like, this is awful. It's embarrassing. So then it was like, I gotta get my shit together.

WINE MOMS

As discussed in chapter 3, drinking is undergoing a process of normalization among women. This appears to include mothers. A striking example is the popularity of the term "wine mom." Although not exactly scientific, there are definitions out there. Ashley Fetters of *The Atlantic* defines a "wine mom" as "someone who likes a drink to take the edge off parenting, and who's willing to poke fun at that fact."[29] The wine mom concept emerged in the mid-2010s and spread rapidly through social media in the form of jokes, memes, and viral videos. The following are typical: "The most expensive part of having kids is all the wine you have to drink." "Wine is to moms what duct tape is to dads. It fixes everything." "It's mom's turn to wine." I asked participants whether they had ever heard the terms "wine mom," "mommy juice," or "mommy drinking culture" and what those terms mean to them. Most had. "Wine moms are soccer moms that take the Starbucks cup to the game and they're loaded up with whatever concoction." "The mom who always has a glass with her, is always trying to make everything a party and everyone have a drink!" "On television and stuff it seems like ladies are always drinking wine and the 'mom' wine and that sort of stuff." "I know tons of women who do, like, kind of have that 'wine thing.'" "It's always like, the 'women and wine.' Like, your child is so hard to deal with you have to drink to deal with it. That type of thing? I've seen that. Yeah. I've felt that. There's a Facebook group called Unfiltered Moms or something like that. Something like that is what they would post."

SUSAN: There's a term called "wine mom." Have you heard that?

KIM: I have.

SUSAN: So what does that mean to you?

KIM: Just a mom's way to get together and release steam. You always see those cups about surviving motherhood "one sip at a time" or something like that. I relate that more to coffee. I'm a coffee mom.

NADINE: I think more how it's kind of become like a hip thing, like trendy to kind of be, you know, like women and wine. You hear all those kinds of like fun kitschy little event things. I think that they're kind of trying to make it more acceptable for women to drink almost.

JOELLYN: I definitely think there's a cultural association with women and wine and with motherhood and wine, and there's all these memes and jokes and T-shirts, and a million different things out there saying like, oh, you know, moms need wine, all moms drink wine. It's like a bombardment of messages about, this is what moms do.

The popular Facebook group Moms Who Need Wine calls itself a "medical company" and has on its main page, inexplicably, a picture of Homer Simpson passed out and drooling. There are many websites and blogs of this nature, such as Mommy Needs a Cocktail, or the even more direct, WineMom. Leigh explained, "I think there's a lot of the new culture of, like, mommies and their drinks. And I think it's kind of hard to escape from that, given the amount of memes and things one sees posted on Facebook or that people are sharing in their groups." Lori also remarked on how drinking has become a normal and expected activity for mothers: "I guess it's like this idea that it's common to like, *need* to drink, to get through your life with small children and that it's socially acceptable and almost like weird *not* to engage in that kind of activity. Christine said this:

> CHRISTINE: I certainly notice that there's a cornerstone of "mom culture" "mommy juice," that it's acceptable to drink a lot of wine to deal with one's difficult role as a mother. And that isn't stigmatized in the same way that other substance use would be. There's, like, T-shirts, you know, and, like, wine bags. And it's sort of odd . . . I don't know that I think that it's bad or good. It's just very prevalent, as long as it's wine.

According to historian Lisa Jacobson, wine-mom humor "allows women to embrace their identities as mothers, while also refusing to be solely defined by their role . . . and are candid expressions of frustration at the somehow simultaneous monotony and chaos of modern mothering."[30]

WINE AND TARGET

As was discussed in chapter 4, I asked participants about wine-related products they may have seen, what I refer to as "wine swag."

> HANNAH: I would say wine and drinking is a common gift amongst my friends we get for each other, like new wine glasses, or like a wine cooler thing. That was a recent gift that I got. So, yeah, I mean I think that "wine and Target" is popular. Like, if you're a mom you do "wine and Target."
>
> SUSAN: What's wine and Target?
>
> HANNAH: So, like, if you're a mom, you like wine. If you're a mom, you go to Target. It's just, like, a perception.

Learning about "wine and Target" led me down an unexpected and rather disturbing path—products being designed and/or marketed to encourage drinking among mothers. The most notable is Pedialyte, a liquid medicine used to rehydrate sick children and a staple in the medicine cabinet of American parents. It seems that Pedialyte as a remedy for hangovers has been an open secret among the soccer mom set for many years. When I spied a joint Pedialyte/Coors Light display in the liquor section of my local grocery store, I saw this was no rumor. It turns out that in 2018, the use of Pedialyte for this purpose was outed in a series of articles, such as "Pedialyte Is the Hottest

Hangover Cure, but Does It Really Work?," "Pedialyte and Other Good Ways to Bounce Back from a Hangover," and "How Pedialyte Got Pedialit."[31] Pedialyte capitalized on this market and created a series of products specifically for adults (e.g., Pedialyte Sparkling Rush Powder Packs), but it was clear that mothers were their target market given that these products are located in the baby sections of Walmart and Target. Moreover, Pedialyte engaged in a massive social media campaign (#teampedialyte) and sent St. Patrick's Day and New Year's Eve care packages to followers. Pedialyte marketed itself as "a fizzy way to quickly replenish fluids and electrolytes lost to dehydration." Pedialyte's own website once read, "Hangovers are the worst. If you've had one, you know there's no quick fix. Pedialyte is not a hangover cure, but it can help with the dehydration you may experience after a couple of cocktails. So rehydrate with Pedialyte to feel better fast." Any mention of hangovers has since been removed from the website and replaced with general information on dehydration.[32] However, Pedialyte as a hangover cure is still being promoted by celebrities and social media influencers such as Cardi B.

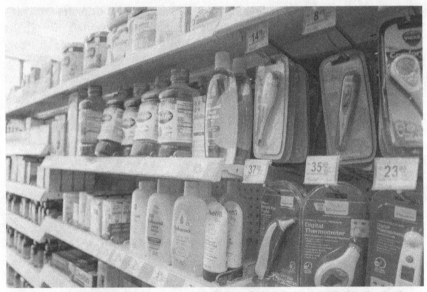

Pedialyte, a rehydration product designed for children, is now being marketed to adults. *Source:* Gado Images/Alamy Stock Photo, Image ID: KGJ34T

There is now a wide range of products that normalize, if not encourage, drinking among mothers. High Key Wine Pouches, designed to look like Capri Sun juice pouches, are "portable and discreet." Julie Scagell writes in her article on Scary Mommy, "Someone Invented Wine Juice Boxes Because We

Deserve to Be Happy," "If your kid plays sports, you know it can get hot out and as the afternoon drags on (and on, and on), why not give yourself a hand by pulling one of these out of your cooler? Just twist open the cap, find the built-in straw, and their game just got *a lot* more interesting."[32] The culture of wine and Target even showed up in a recent *Saturday Night Live* sketch in which a group of women gathered for a birthday party. Out of every gift bag came a kitschy sign. Things started out harmless enough ("Wine Gets Better with Age. I Get Better with Wine") but quickly took a dark turn ("I Put Wine Bottles in Other People's Recycling Bins so the Garbage Men Won't Know How Much I Go Through in a Week," and "Hey Barkeep, I Wanna Die Tonight." The skit was the subject of a great deal of media attention and numerous articles, suggesting it hit close to home.

MOTHERS BEHAVING BADLY

Women, especially mothers, are expected to be "the moral guardians of the family" who must always maintain control.[33] Women who drink have at various points in history been considered "misbehaving women." Recall the "flappers" of the 1920s and "Girls Just Want to Have Fun"–type drinking among young women in the 1980s. Sociologist Jo Littler examined representations of mothers increasingly present in the media, which she refers to as *mothers behaving badly* (MBB). She defines the social type of MBB as "first, mothers in the midst of highly chaotic everyday spaces where any smooth routine of domesticity is conspicuous by its absence; and second, mothers behaving hedonistically, usually through drinking and partying, behavior that is more conventionally associated with men or women without children."[34] She is careful to point out that MBB is reserved for privileged women. Poor mothers, mothers of color, and especially mothers receiving public assistance are not afforded this same luxury. Like wine moms, mothers behaving badly are not *truly* bad. A participant in my study, Megan, said, "When I think of a movie like *Bad Moms*, they just drink themselves silly. But it's like, they've had it. They're at the end of their rope." Movies like *Bad Moms* and *Bad Moms Christmas* portray women rejecting impossible standards of motherhood in favor of behaviors the exact opposite—drinking, smoking, drugs, and sex.

BRENDA: A couple weeks ago I went to a show of two comedic women. Their website is #IMOMSOHARD. They're hilarious and their videos are hilarious and a lot of the videos that they have posted don't necessarily involve alcohol, but I was struck in the show that one of the moms through the entire thing had a glass of wine. And she had it in her hand a lot. And it was kind of a crutch, like, she would get to say something sassy because she had a glass of wine . . . kind of that, you know, sort of attitude. When I was watching it, I was like, you know the other lady is *hilarious* and she's hilarious with her physical comedy and she's got kind of a wicked edge to her comedy. And she wasn't drinking. Didn't use that crutch. And the other lady did.

SUSAN: Were there any jokes about alcohol in the show?

BRENDA: Oh yeah! Just about, you know, sometimes moms need a little something, that kind of joke. Yeah. That, and they were making it a big celebratory atmosphere, like "You got out of the house! This is great! We're gonna have a girls' night!"

A *ladette* is a young woman who takes part in "laddish behavior"—or as the *Oxford English Dictionary* puts it, "young women who behave in a boisterously assertive or crude manner and engage in heavy drinking sessions."[35] Author Lucy Rocca, in her book *The Sober Revolution: Women Calling Time on Wine O'Clock*, states, "For me, coming of age during the 'ladette' years when it was suddenly de rigueur to neck pints on a night out in an effort to keep up with the lads, meant that my lack of awareness in recognizing when I'd had enough to drink, and my desire to consume alcohol to the point of collapse, both went largely unnoticed."[36] According to Emelda Whelehan, "the ladette offers the most shallow model of gender equality; it suggests that women could or should adopt the most anti-social and pointless of 'male' behavior as a sign of empowerment."[37] Many of my participants did not buy it either.

BONNIE: I think it's unfortunate that they have to do that. It's like you can't get through one, two-hour time span without having a drink.

SHARON: I've got a friend who's considerably younger than I am. I've gotten to know her because she has two autistic boys. She's in a horrible situation. Single mom, recent, ugly divorce. And I know that about once a week, she gets someone to take the kids and drinks a lot. And it worries me. Just because I know that she's in a really tenuous situation, and that if it became problem drinking, there's four little boys, and two of them who are disabled, who can't afford to have their mom impaired in any way. And you know, that worries me.

SUSAN: Have you ever talked to your friend about it at all?

SHARON: She's really super-sensitive about it. And she told me at the time, "I know I'm drinking too much. I'm coming home every night and having a six pack of beer. I know I'm drinking too much," but it's the way she talks about it.

Although parental alcohol use disorders are associated with child abuse and neglect, mothers engage in numerous strategies to minimize harm to their children. A thirty-seven-year-old mother in Pamela Raine's study of women who had been in treatment said, "I didn't drink through the day because I had a baby and school but at nighttime that's when it increased, or probably weekends where somebody else could look after her."[38] Other women waited until their children were in bed or waited until they had someone to look after the kids or were out of the house. Many of my participants felt strongly about not drinking in front of children.

> PARKER: If you're talking about women who may be feeling that need to cope and using alcohol to do it, it's probably the pressure of having to do everything right. All the time. And having that coming from a boss and having that coming from a spouse or having that feeling of I need to be a good mom, but now the kids are in bed and I can do this thing that makes me feel good. And it's quick.

SOBER MOTHERS

Although empirical research is scarce, news stories suggest the tide may be turning against the mommy drinking culture. Model Chrissy Teigen, mother of two and wife of singer John Legend, unexpectedly told fans in an Instagram post that she's "four weeks sober." She said she was inspired by the book *Quit Like a Woman: The Radical Choice Not to Drink in a Culture Obsessed with Alcohol*, by Holly Whitaker.[39] In an article in *Harper's Bazaar*, actress Anne Hathaway, who had at the time a three-year-old son, declared she's giving up alcohol for eighteen years. She said she "plans to take up drinking again once her son goes off to college: 'I'm going to move to a vineyard and spend the back half of my life completely sloshed, happy, sun-drenched. That's the plan!'"[40] Articles and essays about women and drinking have become increasingly dark. Scary Mommy has recently published numerous articles about the seriousness of drinking among mothers, such as "The Uneventful Monday Night That Made Me Stop Drinking." The author, who describes herself as "a successful and highly motivated businesswoman, wife, and mom," found herself regularly drinking two, three, or four glasses of wine sitting on the couch watching Netflix and became worried about her method of "self-care."[41] There are now as many articles critical of mommy wine culture as supportive of it: "Giving Up Alcohol Has Given Me My Mojo Back," and "Let's Normalize Non-Alcoholic Offerings at Parties and Events," and "I'm Sober and Working to Shed the Shame of Alcoholism," and "My Name Is Mommy, and I'm an Alcoholic."

Indeed, children can serve as strong motivation for women to drink less. In a study by Bohrman et al., one of only a few qualitative studies of women and alcohol, a participant said, "The only way to change it is to change my behav-

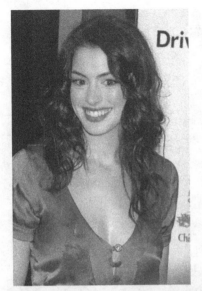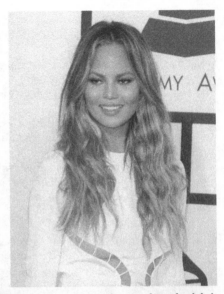

Mothers Anne Hathaway and Chrissy Teigen are among a growing number of celebrities who have publicly discussed quitting alcohol. *Source left*: Everett Collection, Inc./ Alamy Stock Photos, Image ID: C63KNB. *Source right*: WENN Rights, Ltd./Alamy Stock Photo, Image ID: #ETFBH3

ior and I didn't really wanna face that, but it's getting to a point where I got to because I have a child that depends on me."[42] Mothers have begun writing about their struggles with alcohol on public platforms. A 2021 Google search of "mommy wine culture" yielded 3.8 *million* results. "Being a Heavy-Drinking 'Bad Mom' Is More Worrisome than Funny," "That Wine O'Clock' Sh*t Is Cute and All, but It Hurts Real People," and as Ashley Abramson writes in the *Washington Post*, "The cheeky 'wine mom' trope isn't just dumb. It's dangerous." She tells about her own experience: "Some nights I had just a glass. Other nights, depending on my level of despair and boredom, it was an entire bottle. On days when the trenches of early motherhood were particularly condemning and isolating, my nightly wine ritual gave me a break—an escape—from the sticky, cluttered, anxious life I had pieced together as a new mother."[43] Journalist Nicole Pelletiere spoke with a number of reformed wine-moms for her article, "'A Pump-and-Dump Kind of Day': How Wine-Mom Culture Shifted from Funny Memes to Unhappy Hangovers," one of whom had been drinking a bottle of wine nightly. That mother said, "I needed an outlet and I needed a way to escape. It seemed like a perfectly healthy and almost chic way to decompress. I knew a lot of my friends were doing the same thing."[44] Martha Carucci, author of the book *Sobrietease*, provides a gripping account of her own experiences in "The Soccer Mom Next Door" (see box).[45]

THE SOCCER MOM NEXT DOOR

For many, the word "alcoholic" conjures up images of a vagabond on the street drinking from a brown paper bag. But what about the mom sitting next to you at the PTA meeting or in the stands at your child's soccer game? I was that mom.

I drank to numb. I drank to escape. I drank to celebrate, mourn, relax, and to feel better. Name an occasion and I drank to it, for it, because of it. It was a way of everyday life. I knew no other way. What started out as fun, social drinking turned into an absolute necessity. My life was falling apart around me, but I continued to drink. There was no way I was an alcoholic. Not me— an Ivy League–educated, upper-middle class lobbyist and suburban mother of three.

I didn't see anything wrong with the way I was living. I thought it was normal. Like my friends, I thought I "deserved" that drink at the end of a stressful day taking care of the kids. Why wouldn't I bring a stroller full of wine and beer out trick-or-treating with my kids on Halloween? Or celebrate Arbor Day with rounds of shots?

It was fun. And funny at times. And "normal" according to the messages society gave me. Until it wasn't. Until my hands shook from withdrawal until I could get alcohol back into my system. Until alcohol completely took over my life, and my life became unmanageable. Until my kids no longer had a mom who was present and functioning, but spent her days and nights either intoxicated or massively hung over. My life was spiraling rapidly out of control and alcohol took me to a very, very dark place.

I am one of the lucky ones. I found a way out. I got help. I work hard every day to stay sober and be present for my family and friends and try to share my experience, strength and hope with others.

—Martha Carucci,
blogger and author of *Sobrietease*
(www.sobrietease.wordpress.com)

CONCLUSION

Women's use of alcohol varies across the lifecourse, typically peaking in young adulthood and declining with age. Mothers traditionally drink less alcohol than women without children, especially when there are young children in the home. However, alcohol consumption does appear to be increasing among mothers. This chapter provides some reasons why: Keeping up with the boys at work, unrelenting housework, intensive mothering, and the loss of freedom that comes with having children, bolstered by a wine mom culture that makes it all okay. In an environment where most mothers have limited ability to go to the gym, get a massage, read, or have anything resembling a personal life, alcohol has become an accessible and reliable form of "self-care" for mothers. Without a social safety net and embedded in a competitive parenting culture, American mothers toil away on their own, ashamed to ask for help. Mothers who come to perceive themselves as having trouble with alcohol are reluctant to tell anyone, because to do so means admitting to being a "bad mom," which, unlike in the movies, has real consequences such as loss of custody. There are few outpatient programs for women and few A.A. groups geared toward women rather than men, and most groups do not welcome children or offer childcare. Unable to discuss real problems, especially in the shiny world of social media, women commiserate through memes, jokes, and gag gifts. Hilarious. Meanwhile, an ever-increasing array of products is capitalizing on their struggles. But there is more. In chapter 6, I discuss some findings regarding how women are affected by not just their own use of alcohol, but the use of alcohol among important people in their lives.

Chapter Six

Ripple Effect

TRACY: Alcohol has impacted my life in ways that I could have never imagined. And my husband's ex-wife is not *my* ex. She is like two degrees of separation from me. And it has caused so many problems. My husband and I joke, she's the gift that keeps on giving.

—Tracy, age 36, married, one biological child and two stepchildren

I was not prepared for the extent to which my participants wanted to talk about *other people*. In this chapter, I describe how women's relationships and well-being are influenced by the drinking behavior of others. As Kenneth Leonard and Rina Eiden state, "Alcohol use is often part of the fabric of marriage and family life."[1] Recall from chapter 1 that ecological theory emphasizes the family as a whole and how family members, and relationships between family members, are intertwined. For example, women drink more when they perceive approval from people important to them, and their level and pattern of alcohol consumption tends to match that of partners, family, and friends. Women with a biological family member who has had problems with alcohol are significantly more likely to drink than are other women.[2]

While the majority of participants themselves did not report trouble with alcohol and considered themselves "social drinkers," nearly every participant regardless of their demographic characteristics and background reported alcohol-related problems among close family, extended family, friends, and/or acquaintances. Women's core selves are intimately connected to the roles they occupy vis-à-vis others, as a wife or partner, parent, coworker, friend, and extended family member. Women are referred to as the family "kin keeper" and assume responsibility for maintaining relationships among family members.[3] Knowing this, I shouldn't have been surprised that the participants spent a good portion of their time storytelling. While they were fascinating, I asked myself why these stories mattered in terms of the goals of my study. I quickly saw that they matter because the consequences of family members' and friends' drinking are still *theirs to bear*. Sela's sister struggled her whole life with drugs and alcohol. After she passed away at age thirty-five as a result of alcoholism, Sela and her husband took guardianship of her kids.

> SELA: When she was eighteen she got pregnant with her first child, and she had the two boys eleven months apart. She'd be clean for awhile and then she'd go back. I think she started drinking probably after the boys were born, probably in her mid-twenties, because it was more socially acceptable [than drugs]. She kept a lot of diaries and I went through some of them to kind of piece everything together. She has a lot of writing about drinking at night to just try to cope with all of the anxiety that she felt. But she never found the right help or perhaps wasn't focused or diligent enough to continue to try to fight for the right help. I think she was a little scatterbrained from having two young kids. She's a single mom and she was trying to work her way through school. She worked her butt off. And it got to a point where it was just too much for her.

All the participants described substantial "family drama" resulting from alcohol, and many described a personally painful period stemming drinking, mostly on the part of others. *Family drama* is a commonly understood term and part of our vernacular, but it is rarely found in the scientific literature. In the absence of clear guidance, I define *family drama* as the intermittent, yet chronic, imposition of negative situations and pressures of some family members onto others, or onto one another. Family drama is distinct from everyday stresses and strains in its intensity and destructiveness to relationships and livelihoods.

Family drama can hold people back from completing their education, forming stable relationships, marriage, and simply leading an otherwise tranquil existence. A participant in Casey Bohrman and colleagues' study of low-income mothers said, "My great-grandmother passed away and everything, and they needed me to come back. I had to leave a job that I liked and everything so it wasn't like I wanted to go back because it kinda looked like things were OK." Another said, "I have two best friends and they're both guys. They're needy, like a mutha'. Women don't realize how needy men are. Men are so freakin' needy. It's ridiculous. So it's like at the end of the day I'm a superwoman."[3]

High-drama families cross over the threshold of "troubled families" when issues become known to people and institutions outside the family and require some form of intervention by teachers, social service agencies, and/or law enforcement.[4] Participants told many stories along these lines: "I have some cousins on my dad's side some of whom are now in recovery and it'd be more

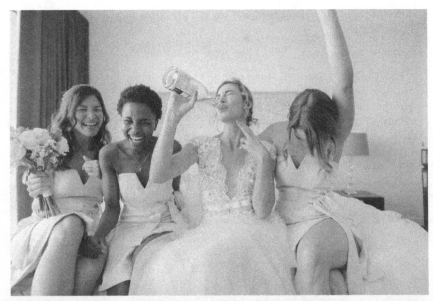

High levels of alcohol consumption at weddings make them prime venues for family drama. *Source*: Jacob Lund/Alamy Stock Photo, Image ID:KXC1FK

my mom saying, 'Oh, did you hear that [cousin] got another DUI?'" "I think the stepdaughter of my friend is now in jail after so many DUIs." Melanie talks about when her daughter went through some difficulties during college:

MELANIE: She graduated, came back to town, started dating a guy and that did not go well. And so she got picked up for a DUI.

SUSAN: She got picked up for a DUI, okay.

MELANIE: Because they broke up and she was just devastated and she started drinking at night and got picked up. But it was a good thing because it taught . . . Dad and I were out of town, so we had to come back to get her out of the police.

SUSAN: How long had she been doing that? Just since the break-up?

MELANIE: She was living at home. She'd been drinking pretty good with this group when she came back home. So I did see heavier drinking, but when she broke up with him, it devastated her. She wasn't a dater. So that was the first boyfriend and then to be, well, I guess they didn't put her in jail, but to be taken down like that . . .

Carly tells the story of her aunt:

CARLY: My mother has a brother—my uncle's ex-wife was an alcoholic. They had five kids. And there's a cousin my age, she's twenty-seven. Back then, she was almost like the parent, and we saw that because they lived with my grandparents.

SUSAN: What happened with them—your cousins and their mom?

CARLY: Their mom went to jail after the third DUI. They grew up with my grandparents until my uncle got situated. And then the oldest . . . actually my grandpa had cancer and he was stealing his pain meds. Didn't end well, like, it ruined so many lives.

Participants were surprisingly sympathetic, I felt, toward drama-prone family members and friends, and typically attributed their behavior to poor mental health, relationship problems, periods of extreme stress, trauma, neglect, and physical and emotional abuse. Nevertheless, participants were protective of their personal well-being.

TOXICITY AND ESTRANGEMENT

There is a shared set of expectations as to how family members are supposed to behave toward one another—unconditionally loving and emotionally close with bonds that are permanent, involuntary, and virtually impossible to dissolve.[5] This is not always possible, and a number of participants told of relationships made "toxic" as a result of alcohol. They managed this by minimizing their dealings with troublesome family members (or friends) or cutting them off completely. Some had read one of the many self-help books on maintaining "healthy boundaries" such as *Surviving the Toxic Family*, *Co-dependent No More*, and *Emotionally Immature Parents*. Some had received counseling. Others simply had an epiphany that they were "done." Having firm boundaries as to what behavior a person is willing to tolerate on the part of others is important to one's emotional health. For example, ambiguity in family boundaries, having family members who are "there but not there," appear in one's life sporadically, or are unreliable sources of support is associated with chronic stress.[6] Family members who continually strain boundaries, and the emotional exhaustion created by difficult relationships, often leads to *estrangement*. Estrangement has been defined in different ways. Researcher, educator, and social worker Kylie Agllias says this:

Family estrangement is generally defined as a reaction to intense emotion or conflict resulting in the distancing or loss of affection between one or more members of a family, where at least one party is dissatisfied with the situation. When family members stop speaking and when they stop contact, this is termed *physical estrangement*. When family members have infrequent, perfunctory, and often uncomfortable contact, this is termed *emotional estrangement*. People who are emotionally estranged often compare family interactions to "walking on eggshells." A person might actively pursue estrangement from family members because it "provides relief and space to heal from a difficult relationship."[7]

Estrangement is associated with anxiety, grief, loss, isolation, and stigma, although it may have positive effects of personal growth, healing, and developing firmer boundaries.[8] Alcohol and drug use are among factors associated with estrangement among adult family members, particularly between parents and children.[9] A number of participants described estrangement in their own families that they saw as caused, at least in part, by alcohol. Ginny was estranged from her mother.

> GINNY: My mom is a hardcore alcoholic and a toxic human being. Her mom's [Ginny's grandmother] a hardcore alcoholic and still alive. It's like, God damn, guys, how the fuck do you drink this much and you're not, like, dead? [laughs] I mean, she drinks, like, half a bottle of rum, like, every day. But I don't think that's only where the negative resides, because I have a lot of alcoholics in my family.
>
> SUSAN: On one side or both?
>
> GINNY: Both. Everywhere. I think because there's so much rampant alcohol abuse as a crutch to deal with mental issues and just like, not feeling worthy as a human being because your parents sucked. I mean, you can look back through history and be like, "Great-grandfather! You caused a lot of this shit that I still have to deal with—fuck you! Like, you're just a total trash human being. You made this, and my mom totally sucked." I think because it's all family, I'm just kind of like, okay, well, I'm stuck with you.

Alcohol is generally just one among many factors leading to estrangement, as was the case for Melanie. "My parents' divorce happened while I was away at college. So when I came back, my dad was really bad. So I didn't see him as much. I maintained a relationship with him, and a good relationship. I felt bad for him. He was a wonderful dad. But he just got caught up in this drinking and couldn't control it." Hannah's parents also divorced:

> HANNAH: It was absolutely the case that their marriage fell apart because of alcohol. I know that she tried to get him into rehab and I know that he went once and as soon as he came back, he didn't stop.
>
> SUSAN: And do you see him? Did you see him after your parents separated?
>
> HANNAH: Growing up we saw him weekends and Wednesdays. I don't see him anymore. I don't have anything to do with him anymore.
>
> SUSAN: Is it because of something he's done? Or just his behavior?

HANNAH: You can't go there on a Friday and expect to have a conversation with him. And you can't go there any time before noon on Saturday or Sunday. My son was born and he's never met him. He's one of those people that when I talk about alcoholics who turn away from people in their lives—he's done that to us. He prioritizes the people that will come to his shop and party with him. That's just not us and so we didn't get prioritized. He prioritizes my stepmom and her kids who will go there and smoke weed and drink until four a.m.

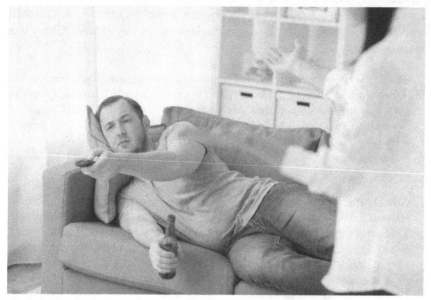

Alcohol overuse is a well-known contributor to poor interpersonal relationships. *Source*: Lev Dolgachov/Alamy Stock Photo, Image ID: JK44JW

A rift with one family member inevitably seeps into relationships with non-estranged family members resulting in "secondary estrangement."[10] This was the case in Diane's family, whose mother she describes as an alcoholic.

DIANE: We all kind of tiptoe around my sister because she is *explosive* in terms of her personality. And the last time my sister and I had an argument, which was, like, literally over nothing, she didn't talk to me for two years and it was *hell*. So, everybody has kind of a fear of my sister in terms of how she'll react to things. I've had better conversations [about my mom] with my brother and he's kind of a soft heart.

Tracy talks about her stepdaughter:

TRACY: She was diagnosed with bipolar. I think she has personality disorder. She writes a mental health blog about the struggles of being in college.

SUSAN: That sounds like a good outlet for her.

TRACY: I brought it up the last time she tried to commit suicide. I said, "You've got to find another outlet because you're taking one extra depression pill, checking yourself into the hospital to get your stomach pumped. That's attention seeking. You're not actually trying. We both know a bottle of Tylenol will do the trick." So my husband is to the point where he doesn't respond anymore, which I think was a great move on his part.

Parents' relationships with their children are often mixed, and relationships with stepchildren tend to be more negative than with biological children. However, poor relationships with one child can negatively affect relationships with other children and hurt parents' well-being overall.[11]

In contrast to family relationships, friendships are voluntary relationships that encompass intimacy, equality, and shared interests, provide important sources of support, and are positively associated with well-being across the lifecourse and can be as important as relationships with family.[12] Several participants discussed how alcohol strained friendships to the point that the relationship dissolved:

GLENDA: I had a friend whose grandma died and was important to him and he turned to alcohol as a coping mechanism. This person used to be super outgoing, loved doing things other than sitting at home and drinking. Like on a weekend we would go on a hike with our dogs. After he started drinking, no. Not anymore. The only thing he wanted to do was be somewhere where he could drink.

SUSAN: Do you know what happened to him?

GLENDA: I don't. He just became extremely toxic and it was best to distance myself, not because I thought I was going to do the same thing but his energy drained mine and I got tired of phone calls at three o'clock in the morning, you know, saying, "Come get me from ABC and D," you know? Props to him for calling me, but it became a problem where it was like, should I just stay up today till three in the morning? Should I just meet you there somewhere? Can we get this earlier? It was like no. It was always drinking.

GINNY: The one friend I did have who is an alcoholic, I told her she's an alcoholic. She was just drinking and drinking and drinking and I'm like, "I kinda think that maybe you shouldn't do that. You're not drinking socially anymore. You're not having a drink *with* us. You're drunk every morning when I come downstairs. You have a master's degree. So I think you're not sorting through some things, and I think you should probably do that rather than just get hammered by yourself every night." She stopped talking to me for like a year, but now she's in A.A., and she told me a year and a half ago, "I'm sorry I was a dick. You told me you thought I had a problem, but I just wasn't really in a space to hear that," and I'm like, "It's fine. I kinda felt like you needed to hear it, which is why I said it at the risk of you not talking to me anymore."

Tracy talks about her old friend.

> TRACY: And then she didn't drink for six months and then we saw each other at
> our pool and just started talking again. And now our friendship is very close, but
> it has gotten to the point where now when we get together it's always around.
>
> SUSAN: So she's drinking again.
>
> TRACY: She's drinking again. Not as much as me. When she drinks, it is so
> humiliating to be around her. I just can't do it.
>
> SUSAN: Because she behaves . . .
>
> TRACY: I have told her about her behavior and she has cried from shame and
> embarrassment. She's the girl that dumps her purse in the middle of the bar in
> a tantrum. It's just embarrassing going out to eat with her even after probably
> two or three drinks. It's embarrassing. I'm no longer able to meet her for happy
> hour, things like that, and most importantly, I don't want to.

IT'S NOT ME, IT'S YOU

Othering is the process of "interpersonal differentiation" whereby a dominant group or person uses negative attributes to distinguish others from
themselves.[13] Originally developed to understand subordination of women
and people of color, othering involves elevating one's own values, standards,
and behavior over others. For example, in a study of women provided with
health advice on the links between alcohol and breast cancer, all considered
themselves "normal" drinkers and therefore set aside alcohol's risk to health
as irrelevant. Moreover, they considered themselves fundamentally different
from people with an alcohol "problem," which they equated with alcoholism,
loss of control, and severe harm.[14] Othering was not uncommon among the
participants in my study—that they do not, and would never, engage in the
outrageous behavior they've witnessed on the part of others. Kori described
one of her girlfriends:

> KORI: We're silly about it, but we're not [overdoing it], at least with my group
> of friends . . . but I have one friend that gets really sloppy drunk. So I do not go
> out with her. We've had that conversation. I said, it's not safe for you and puts
> me in a bad situation and anybody that's with you when you do that because you
> need to be protected. I remember one of my friends getting married and some-
> one kept buying her drinks, and I found her and this guy was trying to drag her
> out. And I'm like, "Excuse me, uh, thank you, hand her over."

SUSAN: This was the night before her wedding? Where was her fiancé?

KORI: Well, he was off having his own party. So they were both hungover the day of their wedding. I'm sitting there going, why did you both drink to excess the night before your wedding? Because it was something that she had never done prior. We'd go out drinking and she'd have a couple of drinks, but nothing to the extent of sloppy drunk that we had to carry her out to the car.

SUSAN: Is she still a drinker?

KORI: No, she's not. I mean, she's got two kids, one's in college now, so that's not even on the radar. She's doing a lot of things. They ended up being divorced and, I mean, of course everything's in hindsight, you find out things after the fact.

Jennifer "othered" her younger self.

JENNIFER: My stepdad was a really bad alcoholic and had a lot of serious mental health issues. And then my biological father was a drug addict, and my mom is just a fucking mess, so my life was raw. So yeah, I was set up to be a train wreck from day one. So I started drinking at thirteen. Like, as soon as it occurred to me to get out of my house and forget about what was happening there. And then I found alcohol and I was like, I can leave that stress completely for, you know, the three hours a night. Or whatever. So it was like the perfect answer to be right until I got in my twenties where I could drink all the time and it became like, "Oh, this could be a problem." So then you say, "Am I going to quit? Or am I going to just do this socially?" It can't solve my mental health issues. That that's not the answer, but when you're thirteen, it seems like an excellent answer.

Ella was shocked by her husband's family's outrageous drinking and wanted no part of that lifestyle.

ELLA: It could have been a huge deal-breaker in our marriage when I look back on it. He's the youngest of six kids. He comes from a big Catholic family. The more alcohol at events, the better. Baptisms, birthdays, Christmas, holidays. I remember going and his gramma was like ninety-three and the brother-in-law was *hitting on* the gramma. He was so drunk. And I was like, okay, *wow*. And then my husband's other brother was drunk out of his mind. We had conversations when we were first dating about this. I was just super-uncomfortable. Especially seeing weirdness going on. And so we kind of came to a place where we didn't want that stuff going on, so we did not serve alcohol at our kids' baptisms or birthday parties. I have a billion nieces and nephews on that side and they're all getting married now. All of them have been drunk together and they're trying to give speeches and my husband would say, "That is not going to happen at our kids' weddings."

SANDWICHED

Regardless of their marital status or whether or not they have children, most American women have substantial family caregiving responsibilities. For example, millions of women are part of the *sandwich generation*. These are adults, mostly women, who are "sandwiched" between two generations that rely on their care. Most are mothers. More than one in ten (12 percent) mothers with children under eighteen are "multigenerational caregivers," responsible for the care of another adult (e.g., shopping, household chores, financial management, doctor's appointments). Women who are multigenerational caregivers spend forty minutes longer engaged in these duties per day than do men in that same role.[15] These duties take a toll, as was the case with Brenda:

> BRENDA: We are recognizing and we are being recognized by others as having very stressful lives; we're juggling eighteen balls in the air. I'm a sandwich generation, I'm parenting my mom, I'm parenting my kids, and still trying to take care of myself at the end of the day. We have a Jacuzzi bathtub. My husband one time said, "Why do you like taking baths so much?" And I said, "Because it's about a half hour or forty-five minutes where nobody needs me." And if they do, I'm in the tub and I can't hear them.

Women's caretaking responsibilities can start well before adulthood. Children in families with alcohol and drug use are more likely than other children to be "parentified," meaning they are compelled to take on adult responsibilities before they are developmentally mature enough to handle them. Parentification has been linked lower self-worth and behavior problems in adolescence.[16] Melanie and Brenda are examples of parentified children.

> MELANIE: My parents ended up divorced. My dad's alcohol use got progressively worse as he got older to the point that they ended up separating when I was in college. I was so busy with everything. And I knew when I left home, there were issues. Cause I was over there. I'm the oldest, there were siblings at home. And so protecting them from some of the stuff that was beginning to happen.

> BRENDA: I was in seventh grade. My mom started drinking too much. And my dad, he traveled a lot for work, and she would drink at night. I could *hear* the cabinet—there is a specific cabinet where alcohol was kept—and I could hear it close so I knew she was drinking and I was very concerned about it, and actually, as a young kid, I don't know why I did this, I went one day and I marked the bottle that I figured she was drinking out of, and when my dad came home several days later it was down a lot, and I took it to him and I said, "This is what's happening when you're gone, and I don't like it. And I don't want it to keep happening," kind of thing, and he said, "Okay. I'll deal with it." I think it got better for a little while. I'm not even sure I can quantify how much my mom

was drinking after that. I can just tell you what the effects were. And the effects were if you called her by four or five in the afternoon, she was drunk. I live very close to her. I would feel like I had to check on her physically . . . like *go* to the house and check on her if I couldn't get ahold of her, and if I could get ahold of her and I knew that she was drinking.

CONCLUSION

As discussed in chapter 2, alcohol tends to be seen in binary terms: "good" or "bad" and "healthy" or "unhealthy." Families are also generally seen in binary terms: "functional" (marked by stability and absence of problems) versus "dysfunctional" (problematic, not salvageable, and to be avoided). According to Leonard and Eiden, "Alcohol presents two faces to the family. One face is that of a beneficial and healthful beverage that fosters warmth and intimacy. The other face is that of a potentially hazardous potion that jeopardizes one's family through conflict, violence, and deprivation."[17] There are few options for families who sit somewhere in the "in between." Moreover, problematizing heavy drinkers as "trainwrecks" or minimizing heavy drinking as part of women's "crazy college days" discourages open discussion of the wide range of alcohol use patterns families experience. Most families have been touched by alcohol abuse in some way. Rather than being seen as a family issue, alcohol abuse is still largely viewed as an individual failing, and family-level resources are sparse. This approach encourages estrangement. Mothers, sisters, and daughters who struggle with alcohol are at a heightened risk of harm (e.g., poverty, victimization) when cut out of families, and as Lorraine Smith writes in *Alcohol and Alcoholism*, there is a "conspiracy of silence" to protect the female alcoholic, which contributes to the underutilization of the scant services that do exist.[18] Chapter 7 provides a summary of my overall findings and their implications. I have included a discussion of women-led movements that challenge existing narratives pertaining to women's alcohol use. The limitations of the study are discussed, as are future directions for theory and research.

Chapter Seven

Sea Legs

AVA: I bought a house not too long ago. Everything went wrong with the house that could. Leaking roof. Bathrooms leaking. It's a one-hundred-year-old house. I kind of knew what I was getting into, but there is definitely stress with the house. It's like, oh, my God. I can't do anything about it, but I can have a glass of wine.

—Ava, age 25, single, no children

A glass of wine. Can a glass of wine hold the complexity of women's lives? Can a bottle of chardonnay encapsulate all that is modern motherhood? My stated goal in embarking on this project was to understand why women's consumption of alcohol has been increasing.

It is a perplexing question given that this potentially harmful behavior has increased alongside improvements in women's lives, at least in terms of their access to higher education, greater options for employment, and growing equality in earnings. In the absence of social and institutional supports (let alone encouragement) for their efforts, women who move to a strange city, buy a house on their own, divorce their husband, or work in an occupation dominated by men would be feeling stress. Parenting children under these conditions could make anyone lose their shit. If a glass or two of wine in the tub or an occasional girls' night out can prevent this, so be it, right?

Several key themes have emerged from the study. I've always felt that conventional narratives of alcohol and alcoholism don't work particularly well for women. The lack of vocabulary is evidence enough. This limited my participants' ability to describe their own and others' use of alcohol beyond social drinking, on the one hand, and alcoholism on the other. Binge drinking was largely dismissed as adolescent hijinks. Alcoholics Anonymous and twelve-step recovery plans dominated discussions of problem drinking.

Holly Whitaker in her article, "The Patriarchy of Alcoholics Anonymous," says A.A.'s model of breaking down one's ego and encouraging members to "humble themselves, to admit their weaknesses, to shut up and listen" is exactly the opposite of what women, who are already quite adept at following the rules and being quiet, need. She asks, "Are women being served by giving themselves over to a 'higher power' when they are struggling to hang onto the little power they have?"[1]

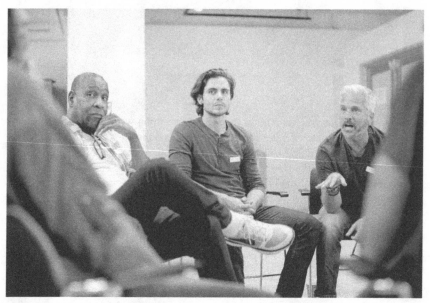

Alcoholics Anonymous and other twelve-step groups were not developed with women's needs in mind. *Source*: MBI/Alamy Stock Photo, Image ID: 2AFGT56

What about the persistence of gender stereotypes? My interviews suggest that women receive very mixed messages about alcohol. Yes, drinking *is* fun and alcohol is instrumental in creating and maintaining cohesiveness among women.[2] Alcohol is also an integral part of religious rituals (e.g., blood of Christ) and celebrations (e.g., champagne at weddings). But, although norms regulating women's drinking have relaxed, women must still navigate an obstacle course of invisible "rules" about what, when, where, and how they drink. The context is pretty limited: one or two "girly" drinks while out with friends, a glass of wine with dinner, a romantic evening with a boyfriend or husband. And most participants held conventional, and gendered, ideas about alcohol, even when coming face to face with behaviors, including their own, that didn't fit these stereotypes.

But if not that, then what? Most memoirs written by women are not un-like those written by men: a downward spiral, hitting rock bottom, the road to recovery, followed by complete abstinence and platitudes about the joys of not drinking. There is no absence of horror stories in these books—DUIs, nasty divorces, custody battles, throwing up on fellow commuters, ruined family celebrations, and even giving birth hungover. Exceptions are few. Two are *Drinking to Distraction* by Jenna Hollenstein and *The Sober Revolution* by Lucy Rocca, in which neither author reached what most would consider "rock bottom."[3] Hollenstein explains she never drove drunk, worked drunk, or injured herself or someone else. Never did she wake up next to a strange man, get fired, go bankrupt, or become homeless. As a result, her efforts were met with resistance: "You don't drink too much; you just worry too much!" Or, "I give you a lot of credit for asking this difficult question. Now how about another round?" And from her mother, "Are you sure you want to do this now? Don't you want to wait until after the New Year?" Nor was she alcoholic enough for the people at A.A. ("You don't understand," and "Maybe you'll get it in a few years"). Rather than expending time convincing others she had a problem, she embarked on her own personal rehab program by asking herself a series of questions such as, "What feelings prompted me to drink?" Similarly, Rocca (who drank two bottles of wine per night before stopping) never considered herself an alcoholic. She says never was her daughter under threat of being taken from her care. She had a nice place to live and never couldn't pay the mortgage, and still looked "reasonably OK." She states, "Pigeonholing very heavy drinkers as 'alcoholics' is an easy way to deflect the accusatory finger away from one's own destructive relationship with booze."[4]

Given the spectrum, continuum, or "gray zone" (whatever you want to call it) along which most women (and men) drink, it makes sense that there be a gray zone of *not* drinking. Rather than an outright rejection of alcohol, a "moderation movement" is underway. This change in thinking is spreading organically through social media. There are numerous Facebook groups that encourage reducing alcohol consumption: *The Alcohol Experiment, Women Who Don't Drink, Soberistas, The Naked Mind*. Drinkers are taking "sober months" (such as "Dry July") to benefit charity or heal their bodies. Many apps have been developed that help monitor drinking and connect with others interested in moderation, such as Dry Days, in which the user tracks their "drinking journey" by logging their daily number of drinks, type of drink consumed, and how they slept and felt upon waking. The app even provides information on dollars saved from not drinking. The potential value of such approaches should not be minimized. Research indicates that treatments that emphasize harm reduction are more effective than those demanding complete abstinence.[5]

As the moral centerpiece of the family, mothers have always been influential in conversations about alcohol, from the temperance movement in the beginning of the twentieth century to the M.A.D.D. movement at the end. Partway into the twenty-first, we're seeing mothers increasingly rejecting the silliness of mom wine culture and taking seriously the negative effects of drinking, not just on their families, but on *themselves*. Rocca writes,

> During the 1990s, feminism for me was best illustrated by the fact that women could happily prop up the bar next to any number of men and smoke and drink pints with them all evening. Now in my late thirties, I consider alcohol to be the key factor in my transformation of my personality from strong and full of gumption in my teens, to depressed, anxiety-ridden, and severely lacking in self-confidence and self-belief in my early thirties—a fine example of *anti-feminism*.[6]

Millennials and Gen-Zers are also pushing back against the rhetoric surrounding women and alcohol. According to cultural historian Lynn Stuart Parramore, the #MeToo movement and movies such as *Promising Young Woman* (in which a woman whose friend committed suicide after being raped gets revenge on "nice guys" who take home and victimize alcohol-impaired women) have "shined a light on alcohol-soaked harassment and assault," encouraging women to reflect on what they are doing to themselves and explore sobriety.[7] In that vein, abstaining from alcohol, getting "sober curious," or "mindful drinking" can be seen as a feminist act. Alongside the moderation movement is a movement to legalize of marijuana. Most participants were supportive of state-level efforts toward legalization and saw its benefits to health, especially in comparison to alcohol. The extent to which women are "switching over" is an important area of inquiry going forward.

Indeed, public policies toward alcohol and other substances are important in shaping attitudes and behavior. Economist Philip Cook says we all "pay the tab" when it comes to the societal impact of alcohol use and abuse.[8] He reviewed the history of alcohol policies in the United States and placed them into two categories. First are policies focusing on "time, place, and circumstance" of drinking (setting a drinking age, employers banning alcohol on the job, regulating where and when alcohol can be sold). The second category focuses on "harm reduction" (making safer roads, making cars more "crashworthy," developing education campaigns, creating more effective treatments). He found that some alcohol policies are more effective than others, such as raising the price of alcohol through excise taxes, which has widespread public approval. Such measures could help reverse the normalization of alcohol by creating a social environment conducive to *not* drinking. However, the multi-billion-dollar liquor industry has a stake in maintaining the "personal responsibility" model of drinking as opposed to a sociological one. Lotta

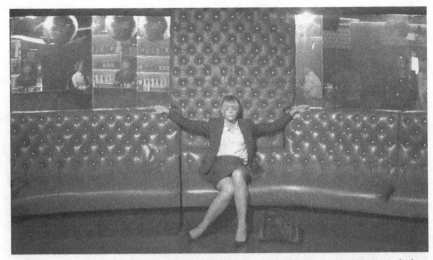

Movies like *Promising Young Woman* are helping to change the narrative around alcohol and victimization. *Source*: Allstar Picture Library Ltd./Alamy Stock Photo, Image ID:2F274KN

Dann (author of *The Wine O'Clock Myth*) discusses the harm being done to the citizens of New Zealand as a result of lobbying by Big Alcohol along with marketing tactics that glorify drinking.[9] The result of these efforts are lax liquor laws, advertising regulations, and sponsorship rules. She says they also deliberately cause confusion by sponsoring wellness events and perpetuate false information about alcohol's risks. However, she is most irritated by how they do not take any responsibility for alcohol's harms by their sole focus on "drinker education," which places the burden of lack of moderation squarely on the shoulders of the consumer. These same "blaming the victim"–type strategies are used to thwart public health advocates' efforts to address threats to public health such as smoking, gambling, and gun violence.

Returning to family systems theory, women don't use alcohol in a vacuum, and the role of alcohol in their lives should be viewed in the context of their relationships. For her book, *Happy Hours*, Devon Jersild interviewed leading experts on women and alcohol, Sharon and Richard Wilsnack. They said women's drinking is closely related to adverse childhood experiences, experiencing a loss, impairment in interpersonal ties, and the expectation that alcohol would make them more self-confident and less sexually inhibited. A fundamental problem with studying women and alcohol is the difficultly in sorting out cause and effect. As Jersild writes, "Most likely, cause and effect work in a reciprocal fashion. Alcohol abuse gets in the way of relationships, but if you are grounded in a sustaining relationship, you aren't as vulnerable to alcohol's pull."[10]

As with all research endeavors, there are limitations to this investigation. Although not the point of the study, one of the main limitations is its lack of generalizability. My sample is based on thirty-two primarily white, hetero-sexual, college-educated women living in the Midwest, and therefore doesn't reflect the experiences of less-educated, lower-income women, women of color, and/or those identifying as LGBTQ+. Research on alcohol use among these groups is sorely lacking and greatly needed. Second, qualitative re-search cannot explicitly test hypotheses, although my findings can help generate them. Additionally, women's recall of previous experiences may be cloudy or inaccurate. I minimized this potential bias by talking to women who were at different stages of life, from younger women right out of college to women with preschool and school-age children to older women whose children have left the nest.

Many of the issues uncovered in this research are not unique to women. One of the most frequent questions I receive with this research is whether I plan to interview men. I do not. For one thing, drinking to *just drink* is a privilege not afforded to women. Women are more likely to use alcohol at home, hide it from others, and drink in ways inconsistent with common understandings of "problem drinking." They may feel they need to drink to keep up with male colleagues. Men are likewise privileged when it comes to the detection and treatment of alcohol problems. Doctors and mental health providers are more likely to brush off heavy alcohol consumption among women, and assessments of alcohol use disorders are geared toward men. Women's heavy consumption of alcohol is trivialized in television, movies, and social media, and "you're a woman, your life sucks, have a drink" mes-saging is everywhere.

Although it is the case that women drink less than men, we should care *more*. Things are changing, but women remain primarily responsible for the care of children and family members. They do most of the household chores. They remember birthdays, shuttle children, do the shopping, and figure out what to have for dinner *every day*. They represent more than 50 percent of the workforce and volunteer their labor as a matter of routine. Women's growing use of alcohol arguably poses a threat to children, families, and society as a whole. But we should care about women not just in terms of what they do for others, but how alcohol is affecting their own hopes and aspirations, even if it is just the right "to party." My findings suggest that more women are drinking more alcohol for lots of reasons: to be more confident, to feel young again, to move up at work, to unwind, and yes, to cope with stress, boredom, and loneliness.

In two large nationally representative samples of Chinese and American adults, quitting drinking was associated with significant improvements in mental health.[11] This research received widespread attention. Should women stop drinking? I can't answer that question or make recommendations as to what a healthy or appropriate amount of alcohol should be. I do think that women should be free to drink, or not, in whatever way suits them and be allowed to chart their own course.

Appendix

Table 1. Characteristics of Interviewees

	Frequency	Percent
Age		
25–29	10	31
30–39	9	28
40–49	8	25
50 and over	5	16
Race and Ethnicity		
White	26	81
Black or African American	2	6
Hispanic	3	9
Asian	1	3
Education		
Some college	5	16
Bachelor's degree	8	25
Graduate or professional degree	19	59
Employment		
Full-time	26	81
Part-time	3	9
Stay-at-home parent	1	3
Not working	1	3
Student	1	3
Occupation		
Research and education	12	38
Administration and communications	9	28
Health and human services	8	25
Business and support services	3	9
Relationship Status		
Single, not currently dating	5	16
Single, dating	1	3

(continued)

Table 1. *(continued)*

	Frequency	Percent
Single, serious romantic partner	4	13
Cohabiting, serious romantic partner	0	0
Married	22	69
Ever Divorced		
Yes	7	22
No	25	78
Number of Children		
0	12	38
1	8	25
2	6	19
3+	6	19
Gender of Children		
No children	12	38
All girls	6	19
All boys	7	22
Mix of girls and boys	7	22
Ages of Children[1]		
5 or younger	9	22
6–12	8	20
13–17	13	32
18–24	6	15
25 and older	5	12
Relationship to Parent[1]		
Biological child	36	88
Adopted child	1	2
Stepchild	2	5
Not reported	2	5
Residence of Children[1]		
In home all of time	31	76
In home part of time	5	12
Outside of home	5	12
Religious Affiliation		
Catholic	5	16
Protestant	8	25
Other	5	16
None	14	44
Religious Service Attendance		
Do not attend	12	38
A few times a year	11	34
Monthly	3	9
Weekly	6	19
Consider Yourself Spiritual Person		
Yes	23	72
No	9	28

(continued)

	Frequency	Percent
Household Income		
Less than $50,000	4	13
$50,000–$74,999	9	28
$75,000–$99,999	6	19
$100,000–$149,999	9	28
$150,000 and more	4	13

Note: Sample consists of 32 participants. Percentages may not add to 100 due to rounding.[1]

Table 2. Alcohol Consumption Patterns of Interviewees (During Last 12 Months)

	Frequency	Percent
Frequency of alcohol consumption		
Less than once a month	4	13
One to three times a month	6	19
Once or twice a week	12	38
Three or more times a week	10	32
Number of drinks on typical day		
1	15	47
2	10	31
3+	7	22
Number of times drank 4+ drinks in two-hour period		
0	15	47
1–11 times in past year	11	34
Once a month or more	6	19
Age at first drink		
6–12	6	19
13–15	8	25
16–18	8	25
19–21	10	32
Have relatives you would consider problem drinkers[1]		
None	6	19
Yes, in immediate family only	5	17
Yes, in extended family only	15	49
Yes, in both immediate and extended family	6	19
Presence of alcohol use disorder[2]		
None	13	41
Mild	15	47
Moderate	4	13
Severe	0	0

Note: Sample consists of 32 participants. Percentages may not add to 100 due to rounding.

Table 3. DSM-5 Criteria for Diagnosing an Alcohol Use Disorder (AUD)

	Yes	No

In the past year, have you:

Had times when you ended up drinking more, or longer, than you intended?

More than once wanted to cut down or stop drinking, or tried to, but couldn't?

Spent a lot of time drinking? Or being sick or getting over the aftereffects?

Wanted a drink so badly you couldn't think of anything else?

Found that drinking—or being sick from drinking—often interfered with taking care of your home or family? Or caused job troubles? Or school problems?

Continued to drink even though it was causing trouble with your family or friends?

Given up or cut back on activities that were important or interesting to you, or gave you pleasure, in order to drink?

More than once gotten into situations while or after drinking that increased your chances of getting hurt (such as driving, swimming, using machinery, walking in a dangerous area, or having unsafe sex)?

Continued to drink even though it was making you feel depressed or anxious or adding to another health problem? Or after having had a memory blackout?

Had to drink much more than you once did to get the effect you want? Or found that your usual number of drinks had much less effect than before?

Found that when the effects of alcohol were wearing off, you had withdrawal symptoms, such as trouble sleeping, shakiness, restlessness, nausea, sweating, a racing heart, or a seizure? Or sensed things that were not there?

Note: The presence of 2 to 3 symptoms is considered a "mild" AUD, 4 to 5 symptoms is considered "moderate," and 6 or more symptoms is considered "severe."

Notes

NOTES ON THE COVID-19 PANDEMIC

1. Stephanie Colbert et al., "COVID–19 and Alcohol in Australia: Industry Changes and Public Health Impacts," *Drug and Alcohol Review* (2020), doi: 10.1111/dar.13092; Leigh Giangreco, "At D.C.'s Liquor Stores, Sales Have Doubled and a Whole Lot of Everclear Is Flying Off the Shelves," accessed July 9, 2020, https://dcist.com/story/20/03/16/at-d-c-s-liquor-stores-sales-have-doubled-and-a-whole-lot-of-everclear-is-flying-off-the-shelves/; Christina C. Ianzito, "Alcohol Use on the Rise During Pandemic," accessed May 22, 2020, https://aarp.org/health/healthy-living/info-2020/coronavirus-alcohol.html; Jonathan S. Zipursky et al., "Alcohol Sales and Alcohol-Related Emergencies During the COVID-19 Pandemic," *Annals of Internal Medicine* (2021), doi: 10.7326/M20-7466.

2. Nielsen, "Rebalancing the 'COVID-19 Effect' on Alcohol Sales," *NielsenIQ*, accessed June 21, 2020, https://www.nielsen.com/us/en/insights/article/2020/rebalancing-the-covid-19-effect-on-alcohol-sales/.

3. Nicholas Biddle et al., "Alcohol Consumption During the COVID-19 Period: May 2020," *Australian National University Center for Social Research and Methods* (2020), accessed June 8, 2021, https://openresearch-repository.anu.edu.au/bitstream/1885/213196/1/Alcohol_consumption_during_the_COVID-19_period.pdf; Daniela Calina et al., "COVID-19 Pandemic and Alcohol Consumption: Impacts and Interconnections," *Toxicology Reports* 8 (2021): 529–35; Michael S. Pollard, Joan S. Tucker, and Harold D. Green, "Changes in Adult Alcohol Use and Consequences During the COVID-19 Pandemic in the US," *JAMA Network Open* 3 (2020): e2022942-e2022942.

4. Susan D. Stewart, "COVID-19, Coronavirus-Related Anxiety, and Changes in Women's Alcohol Use," *Gynecology and Women's Health* (2021), doi: 10.19080/jgwh.2021.21.556057.

5. Ally R. Avery et al., "Stress, Anxiety, and Change in Alcohol Use During the COVID-19 Pandemic: Findings Among Adult Twin Pairs," *Frontiers in Psychiatry*

11 (2020), https://dx.doi.org/10.3389%2Ffpsyt.2020.571084; Julia D. Buckner et al., "Difficulties with Emotion Regulation and Drinking During the COVID-19 Pandemic Among Undergraduates: The Serial Mediation of COVID-Related Distress and Drinking to Cope with the Pandemic," *Cognitive Behaviour Therapy* (2021): 1–15; Silvia Eiken Alpers et al., "Alcohol Consumption During a Pandemic Lockdown Period and Change in Alcohol Consumption Related to Worries and Pandemic Measures," *International Journal of Environmental Research and Public Health* 18 (2021): 1220; William V. Lechner et al., "Increases in Risky Drinking During the COVID-19 Pandemic Assessed via Longitudinal Cohort Design: Associations with Racial Tensions, Financial Distress, Psychological Distress and Virus-Related Fears," *Alcohol and Alcoholism* (2021), doi: 10.1093/alcalc/agab019; Jack Tsai et al., "Psychological Distress and Alcohol Use Disorder During the COVID-19 Era Among Middle- and Low-Income US Adults," *Journal of Affective Disorders* 288 (2021): 41–9.

CHAPTER ONE

1. Gallup, "Alcohol and Drinking," accessed May 20, 2021, https://news.gallup.com/poll/1582/alcohol-drinking.aspx.

2. Herbert Fingarette, *Heavy Drinking: The Myth of Alcoholism as a Disease* (Berkeley, CA: University of California Press, 1988).

3. "Alcoholism" and "alcoholic" as a diagnosis do not and have never appeared in the *Diagnostic and Statistical Manual of Mental Disorders* (the DSM) published by the American Psychiatric Association, now in its fifth edition. There is no agreed-upon definition of either term in the literature and studies routinely contradict the notion that alcoholism is a disease. Rather, research has shown that alcohol overuse and alcohol dependency are the results of a complex set of genetic, physiological, mental, cultural, and social factors. I therefore discourage the use of both terms, aside from my exploration of what these terms mean to the participants in this study and in their own descriptions.

4. Institute of Alcohol Studies, "Changing Trends in Women's Drinking," accessed September 22, 2017, http://www.ias.org.uk/Alcohol-knowledge-centre/Alcohol-and-women/Factsheets/The-effects-of-alcohol-on-women.aspx; OECD, *Tackling Harmful Alcohol Use*, accessed June 10, 2021, https://www.oecd.org/health/tackling-harmful-alcohol-use-9789264181069-en.htm.

5. Marrisa B. Esser et al., "Peer Reviewed: Prevalence of Alcohol Dependence Among US Adult Drinkers, 2009–2011," *Preventing Chronic Disease* 11 (2014), doi: 10.5888%2Fpcd11.140329; Bridget F. Grant et al., "Epidemiology of DSM-5 Alcohol Use Disorder: Results from the National Epidemiologic Survey on Alcohol and Related Conditions III," *JAMA Psychiatry* 72 (2015): 757–66; Richard W. Wilsnack et al., "Gender Differences in Alcohol Consumption and Adverse Drinking Consequences: Cross-Cultural Patterns," *Addiction* 95 (2000): 251–65.

6. Timothy Slade et al., "Birth Cohort Trends in the Global Epidemiology of Alcohol Use and Alcohol-Related Harms in Men and Women: Systematic Review and Metaregression," *BMJ Open* 6 (2016), doi: 10.1136/bmjopen-2016-011827; Aaron

White et al., "Converging Patterns of Alcohol Use and Related Outcomes Among Females and Males in the United States, 2002 to 2012," *Alcoholism: Clinical and Experimental Research* 39 (2015): 1712–26.

7. Bridget F. Grant et al., "Prevalence of 12-Month Alcohol Use, High-Risk Drinking, and DSM-IV Alcohol Use Disorder in the United States, 2001–2002 to 2012–2013: Results from the National Epidemiologic Survey on Alcohol and Related Conditions," *JAMA Psychiatry* 74 (2017): 911–23.

8. Binge drinking is defined by the National Institute of Alcohol Abuse and Alcoholism (NIAAA) as drinking that brings a person's blood alcohol concentration to 0.08 g/dL or higher. This typically occurs when a woman consumes four or more drinks (five or more drinks for men) in about two hours. NIAAA, "Alcohol Facts and Statistics," accessed June 4, 2021, https://www.niaaa.nih.gov/publications/brochures -and-fact-sheets/alcohol-facts-and-statistics; Richard A. Grucza et al., "Trends in Adult Alcohol Use and Binge Drinking in the Early 21st-Century United States: A Meta-Analysis of 6 National Survey Series," *Alcoholism: Clinical and Experimental Research* 42 (2018): 1939–50.

9. Marissa B. Esser et al., "Current and Binge Drinking Among High School Students—United States, 1991–2015," *Morbidity and Mortality Weekly Report* 66 (2017): 474.

10. Sadie Boniface, James Kneale, and Nicola Shelton, "Drinking Pattern Is More Strongly Associated with Under-reporting of Alcohol Consumption Than Socio-Demographic Factors: Evidence from a Mixed-Methods Study," *BMC Public Health* 14 (2014): 1–9; Michael Livingston and Sarah Callinan, "Underreporting in Alcohol Surveys: Whose Drinking Is Underestimated?" *Journal of Studies on Alcohol and Drugs* 76 (2015): 158–64.

11. Joel Achenbach and Dan Keating, "A New Divide in American Death," accessed June 10, 2021, https://www.washingtonpost.com/sf/national/2016/04/10/a-new -divide-in-american-death/?tid=usw_passupdatepg; Allison Aubrey, "With Heavy Drinking on the Rise, How Much Is Too Much?" Accessed September 1, 2017, http://www.npr.org/sections/thesalt/2017/08/16/543965637/women-who-love-wine -are-you-binge-drinking-without-realizing-it.

12. Kennedy Kindy and Dan Keating, "For Women, Heavy Drinking Has Been Normalized. That's Dangerous," accessed August 29, 2017, https://www.washington post.com/national/for-women-heavy-drinking-has-been-normalized-thats-dan gerous/2016/12/23/0e701120-c381-11e6-9578-0054287507db_story.html?utm _term=.6840ab0d9bc2.

13. Claire Nicogossian, "Hoda & Jenna, Please Get Rid of the Wine," accessed January 6, 2021, https://community.today.com/parentingteam/post/hoda-jenna -please-get-rid-of-the-wine; Charlotte Triggs, "Jenna Bush Hager Says Laura Bush Is Not a Fan of Her Today Show Day-Drinking: 'My Mom Judges,'" accessed January 6, 2021. https://people.com/tv/jenna-bush-hager-mom-laura-bush-not-fan-today -show-wine/.

14. Sarah A. Benton, "Caron Study Reveals 'Top 5 Reasons' Mothers Turn to Alcohol," accessed June 11, 2021, https://www.psychologytoday.com/blog/the-high-func tioning-alcoholic/201305/caron-study-reveals-top-5-reasons-mothers-turn-alcohol.

15. Michael R. Frone, "Work Stress and Alcohol Use: Developing and Testing a Biphasic Self-Medication Model," *Work & Stress* 30 (2016): 374–94; Michael R. Frone et al., "Relationship of Work-Family Conflict to Substance Use Among Employed Mothers: The Role of Negative Affect," *Journal of Marriage and the Family* (1994): 1019–30; Michael R. Frone, Marcia Russell, and M. Lynne Cooper, "Relationship of Work–Family Conflict, Gender, and Alcohol Expectancies to Alcohol Use/ Abuse," *Journal of Organizational Behavior* 14 (1993): 545–58; Joseph G. Grzywacz and Nadine F. Marks, "Family, Work, Work–Family Spillover, and Problem Drinking During Midlife," *Journal of Marriage and Family* 62 (2000): 336–48; Helen M. Haydon, Patricia L. Obst, and Ioni Lews, "Beliefs Underlying Women's Intentions to Consume Alcohol," *BMC Women's Health* 16 (2016): 1–12.

16. Sundari Balan et al., "Motherhood, Psychological Risks, and Resources in Relation to Alcohol Use Disorder: Are There Differences Between Black and White Women?" *International Scholarly Research Notices* (2014), doi: 10.1155/2014/437080.

17. Institute of Alcohol Studies, "Why Are Women Drinking More?" Accessed September 22, 2017, http://www.ias.org.uk/Alcohol-knowledge-centre/Alcohol-and -women/Factsheets/Why-are-women-drinking-more.aspx; Kindy and Keating, "For Women, Heavy Drinking Has Been Normalized"; Elisabeth Poorman, "How We Doctors Are Failing Our Patients Who Drink Too Much," accessed June 10, 2021, http:// www.wbur.org/commonhealth/2017/03/31/not-alcholic-drink-heavily.

18. Lynsey K. Romo et al., "An Examination of How Professionals Who Abstain from Alcohol Communicatively Negotiate Their Non-Drinking Identity," *Journal of Applied Communication Research* 43 (2015): 91–111.

19. Kindy and Keating, "For Women, Heavy Drinking Has Been Normalized."

20. Nora Ephron, *I Remember Nothing* (New York: Alfred, 2010), 31.

21. Antonia Abbey and Richard J. Harnish, "Perception of Sexual Intent: The Role of Gender, Alcohol Consumption, and Rape Supportive Attitudes," *Sex Roles* 32 (1995): 297–313; Edith L. Gomberg, "Women and Alcohol: Use and Abuse," *Journal of Nervous and Mental Disease* 181 (1993): 211–19; Antonia C. Lyons and Sara A. Willott, "Alcohol Consumption, Gender Identities and Women's Changing Social Positions," *Sex Roles* 59 (2008): 694–712; Lina A. Ricciardelli et al., "Gender Stereotypes and Drinking Cognitions as Indicators of Moderate and High Risk Drinking Among Young Women and Men," *Drug and Alcohol Dependence* 61 (2001): 129–36.

22. Elvira Elek et al., "Women's Knowledge, Views, and Experiences Regarding Alcohol Use and Pregnancy: Opportunities to Improve Health Messages," *American Journal of Health Education* 44 (2013): 177–90.

23. Claire Gillespie, "Mommy Doesn't Need Wine: The Stigma of Being a Sober Mother," accessed July 18, 2019, https://www.thefix.com/mommy-doesnt-need-wine -stigma-being-sober-mother.

24. Lotta Dann, *The Wine O'Clock Myth* (Sydney, Australia: Allen & Unwin, 2021); Devon Jersild, *Happy Hours: Alcohol in a Woman's Life* (New York: Harper, 2021).

25. Niamh Fitzgerald et al., "Gender Differences in the Impact of Population-Level Alcohol Policy Interventions: Evidence Synthesis of Systematic Reviews," *Addiction* 111 (2016): 1735–47; May Sudhinaraset, Christina Wigglesworth, and David

T. Takeuchi, "Social and Cultural Contexts of Alcohol Use: Influences in a Social–Ecological Framework," *Alcohol Research: Current Reviews* 38 (2016): 35–45.

26. OECD, *Tackling Harmful Alcohol Use.*

27. Gallup, "Alcohol and Drinking."

28. Jeffrey M. Jones, "U.S. Drinkers Divide Between Beer and Wine as Favorite," accessed August 23, 2017, http://www.gallup.com/poll/163787/drinkers-divide-beer-wine-favorite.aspx.

29. Kyle Swartz, "Trends Driving Wine Sales in 2016," accessed June 10, 2021, http://beveragedynamics.com/2016/01/26/9-trends-driving-wine-sales-in-2016/.

30. Emily Heil, "The Key to White Claw's Surging Popularity: Marketing to a Post-Gender World," accessed December 12, 2020, https://www.washingtonpost.com/news/voraciously/wp/2019/09/10/the-key-to-white-claws-surging-popularity-marketing-to-a-post-gender-world/.

31. Alissa Scheller, "Here Are the Rules to Buying Alcohol in Each State's Grocery Stores," accessed June 10, 2021, https://www.huffingtonpost.com/2014/08/26/here-are-all-the-states-t_n_5710135.html.

32. Cheryl Knepper, "Women and the Impact of Addiction: Special Issues in Treatment and Recovery," accessed June 10, 2021, https://www.naatp.org/sites/naatp.org/files/wp-content/uploads/2012/07/Knepper-Women-Presentation.pdf.

33. Swartz, "Trends Driving Wine Sales in 2016."

34. Stacy Briscoe, "Direct-to-Consumer Wine Sales Up $222 Million," accessed December 12, 2020, https://www.winemag.com/2020/08/20/wine-sales-direct-consumer/.

35. Kindy and Keating, "For Women, Heavy Drinking Has Been Normalized."

36. Henneke Hendriks et al., "Picture Me Drinking: Alcohol-Related Posts by Instagram Influencers Popular Among Adolescents and Young Adults," *Frontiers in Psychology* 10 (2020): 2991.

37. GBD 2016 Alcohol Collaborators, "Alcohol Use and Burden for 195 Countries and Territories, 1990–2016: A Systematic Analysis for the Global Burden of Disease Study 2016," *The Lancet* 392 (2018): 1015–35.

38. OECD, *Tackling Harmful Alcohol Use.*

39. Marissa B. Esser et al., "Deaths and Years of Potential Life Lost from Excessive Alcohol Use—United States, 2011–2015," *Morbidity and Mortality Weekly Report* 69 (2020): 1428.

40. NIAAA, "Alcohol Facts and Statistics."

41. Joseph M. Boden and David M. Fergusson, "Alcohol and Depression," *Addiction* 106 (2011): 906–14; Jenny Connor, "Alcohol Consumption as a Cause of Cancer," *Addiction* 112 (2017): 222–28; Samara Joy Nielsen, "Calories Consumed from Alcoholic Beverages by US Adults, 2007–2010," accessed June 11, 2021, https://www.cdc.gov/nchs/products/databriefs/db110.htm; Nicole J. Ridley, Brian Draper, and Adrienne Withall, "Alcohol-Related Dementia: An Update of the Evidence," *Alzheimer's Research & Therapy* 5 (2013): 1–8; Elliot B. Tapper and Neehar D. Parikh, "Mortality Due to Cirrhosis and Liver Cancer in the United States, 1999–2016: Observational Study," *BMJ* 362 (2018), doi: 10.1136/bmj.k2817.

42. Grant et al., "Prevalence of 12-Month Alcohol Use."

43. NIAAA, "Alcohol Facts and Statistics."

44. U.S. Department of Health and Human Services, "Alcohol: A Women's Health Issue," accessed July 10, 2020, https://pubs.niaaa.nih.gov/publications/brochure women/Woman_English.pdf.

45. Jessica L. Mellinger et al., "The High Burden of Alcoholic Cirrhosis in Privately Insured Persons in the United States," *Hepatology* 68 (2018): 872–82.

46. Grant et al., "Epidemiology of DSM-5 Alcohol Use Disorder."

47. Institute of Alcohol Studies, "The Effects of Alcohol on Women," accessed September 22, 2017, http://www.ias.org.uk/Alcohol-knowledge-centre/Alcohol-and -women/Factsheets/Changing-trends-in-womens-drinking.aspx; Jelena Milic et al., "Menopause, Aging, and Alcohol Use Disorders in Women," *Maturitas* 111 (2018): 100–9; Anette Petri et al., "Alcohol Intake, Type of Beverage, and Risk of Breast Cancer in Pre- and Postmenopausal Women," *Alcoholism: Clinical and Experimental Research* 28 (2004): 1084–90.

48. Rosalind A. Breslow et al., "Trends in Alcohol Consumption Among Older Americans: National Health Interview Surveys, 1997 to 2014," *Alcoholism: Clinical and Experimental Research* 41 (2017): 976–86.

49. Aaron M. White et al., "Using Death Certificates to Explore Changes in Alcohol-Related Mortality in the United States, 1999 to 2017," *Alcoholism: Clinical and Experimental Research* 44 (2020): 178–87.

50. Francesco Acciai and Glenn Firebaugh, "Why Did Life Expectancy Decline in the United States in 2015? A Gender-Specific Analysis," *Social Science & Medicine* 190 (2017): 174–80; Ann Case and Angus Deaton, "Rising Morbidity and Mortality in Midlife Among White Non-Hispanic Americans in the 21st Century," *Proceedings of the National Academy of Sciences* 112 (2015): 15078–83; Stephen H. Woolf and Heidi Schoomaker, "Life Expectancy and Mortality Rates in the United States, 1959–2017," *JAMA* 322 (2019): 1996–2016.

51. Knepper, "Women and the Impact of Addiction."

52. Tami L. Mark et al., "Alcohol and Opioid Dependence Medications: Prescription Trends, Overall and by Physician Specialty," *Drug and Alcohol Dependence* 99 (2009): 345–49; Poorman, "How We Doctors Are Failing Our Patients."

53. Gabrielle Glaser, *Her Best Kept Secret* (New York: Simon & Schuster, 2013).

54. John F. Kelly and Bettina B. Hoeppner, "Does Alcoholics Anonymous Work Differently for Men and Women? A Moderated Multiple-Mediation Analysis in a Large Clinical Sample," *Drug and Alcohol Dependence* 130 (2013): 186–93.

55. Pamela Raine, *Women's Perspectives on Drugs and Alcohol: The Vicious Circle* (Farnham, UK: Ashgate Publishing, 2001).

56. Barbara S. McCrady, Elizabeth E. Epstein, and Kathryn F. Fokas, "Treatment Interventions for Women with Alcohol Use Disorder," *Alcohol Research: Current Reviews* 40 (2020), doi: 10.35946%2Farcr.v40.2.08.

57. Gallup, "Alcohol and Drinking."

58. Center for Behavioral Health Statistics and Quality, "More Than 7 Million Children Live with a Parent with Alcohol Problems," accessed July 10, 2021, https://www.samhsa.gov/data/sites/default/files/Spot061ChildrenOfAlcoholics2012 /Spot061ChildrenOfAlcoholics2012.pdf; Rachel N. Lipari and Struther L. Van Horn,

"Children Living with Parents Who Have a Substance Use Disorder," *The CBHSQ Report*, accessed June 5, 2021, https://www.ncbi.nlm.nih.gov/books/NBK464590/.

59. Fe M. Caces et al., "Alcohol Consumption and Divorce Rates in the United States," *Journal of Studies on Alcohol* 60 (1999): 647–52; Raul Caetano, John Schafer, and Carol B. Cunradi, "Alcohol-Related Intimate Partner Violence Among White, Black, and Hispanic Couples in the United States." *Alcohol Research & Health* 25 (2001): 58–65; Shanta R. Dube et al., "Growing Up with Parental Alcohol Abuse: Exposure to Childhood Abuse, Neglect, and Household Dysfunction," *Child Abuse and Neglect* 25 (2001): 1627–40; Grzywacz and Marks, "Family, Work, Work-Family Spillover"; Michael P. Marshal, "For Better or for Worse? The Effects of Alcohol Use on Marital Functioning," *Clinical Psychology Review* 23 (2003): 959–97; Emily N. Neger and Ronald J. Prinz, "Interventions to Address Parenting and Parental Substance Abuse: Conceptual and Methodological Considerations," *Clinical Psychology Review* 39 (2015): 71–82.

60. Gallup, "Alcohol and Drinking."

61. OECD, *Tackling Harmful Alcohol Use*.

62. Jeffrey M. Jones, "Drinking Highest Among Educated Upper-Income Americans," accessed August 23, 2017, http://www.gallup.com/poll/184358/drinking-highest-among-educated-upper-income-americans.aspx; William C. Kerr et al., "Health Risk Factors Associated with Lifetime Abstinence from Alcohol in the 1979 National Longitudinal Survey of Youth Cohort," *Alcoholism: Clinical and Experimental Research* 41 (2017): 388–98.

63. Jones, "Drinking Highest Among Educated Upper-Income Americans."

64. Dan Keating, Kennedy Elliott, and Leslie Shapiro, "White Women Are Dying Faster All Over America—But What About Where You Live?" Accessed September 22, 2017, https://www.washingtonpost.com/graphics/national/death-rates-your-county/.

65. OECD, *Tackling Harmful Alcohol Use*.

66. Jones, "Drinking Highest Among Educated Upper-Income Americans."

67. Grant et al., "Epidemiology of DSM-5 Alcohol Use Disorder"; Bengt O. Muthén and Linda K. Muthén, "The Development of Heavy Drinking and Alcohol-Related Problems from Ages 18 to 37 in a US National Sample," *Journal of Studies on Alcohol* 61 (2000): 290–300.

68. Dan Keating, "Nine Charts That Show How White Women Are Drinking Themselves to Death," accessed July 12, 2021, https://www.washingtonpost.com/news/national/wp/2016/12/23/nine-charts-that-show-how-white-women-are-drinking-themselves-to-death/.

69. Steven H. Woolf, "Changes in Midlife Death Rates Across Racial and Ethnic Groups in the United States: Systematic Analysis of Vital Statistics," *BMJ* 362 (2018), doi: 10.1136/bmj.k3096.

70. Keating, "Nine Charts That Show How White Women Are Drinking Themselves to Death."

71. Susan D. Stewart, Gloria Jones-Johnson, and Cassandra Dorius, "Women and Alcohol Use Over the Lifecourse" (presentation, American Sociological Association, New York, August 10–13, 2019).

72. U.S. Department of Health and Human Services, "Alcohol: A Women's Health Issue."

73. NAAA, *10th Special Report to the US Congress on Alcohol and Health from the Secretary of Health and Human Services*, accessed June 10, 2021, https://pubs .niaaa.nih.gov/publications/10report/10thspecialreport.pdf.

74. Nicole D. Laborde and Christina Mair, "Alcohol Use Patterns Among Postpartum Women," *Maternal and Child Health Journal* 16 (2012): 1810–19.

75. Balan et al., "Motherhood, Psychological Risks, and Resources"; Raul Caetano et al., "The Epidemiology of Drinking Among Women of Child-Bearing Age," *Alcoholism: Clinical and Experimental Research* 30 (2006): 1023–30; Howard D. Chilcoat and Naomi Breslau, "Alcohol Disorders in Young Adulthood: Effects of Transitions into Adult Roles," *Journal of Health and Social Behavior* (1996): 339–49; Ik Young Cho and Kathleen S. Crittenden, "The Impact of Adult Roles on Drinking Among Women in the United States," *Substance Use and Misuse* 41 (2006): 17–34; Grant et al., "Epidemiology of DSM-5 Alcohol Use Disorder"; Fred W. Johnson et al., "Drinking Over the Life Course within Gender and Ethnic Groups: A Hyperparametric Analysis," *Journal of Studies on Alcohol* 59 (1998): 568–80; William C. Kerr et al., "Age-Period-Cohort Modelling of Alcohol Volume and Heavy Drinking Days in the US National Alcohol Surveys: Divergence in Younger and Older Adult Trends," *Addiction* 104 (2009): 27–37; Edith L. Gomberg, "Women and Alcoholism: Psychosocial Issues," *Research Monograph* 16 (1986). 78–120; Carol Miller-Tutzauer, Kenneth E. Leonard, and Michael Windle, "Marriage and Alcohol Use: A Longitudinal Study of 'Maturing Out,'" *Journal of Studies on Alcohol* 52 (1991): 434–40; Laborde and Mair, "Alcohol Use Patterns Among Postpartum Women"; Pamela Mudar, Jill N. Kearns, and Kenneth E. Leonard, "The Transition to Marriage and Changes in Alcohol Involvement Among Black Couples and White Couples," *Journal of Studies on Alcohol* 63 (2002): 568–76; Susan D. Stewart, Gloria Jones-Johnson, and Cassandra Dorius, "Mothers' Alcohol Use When the Children Leave the Nest: An Intersectional Approach" (presentation, Midwest Sociological Society, Chicago, IL, April 17–20, 2019); Andrea L. Stone et al., "Review of Risk and Protective Factors of Substance Use and Problem Use in Emerging Adulthood," *Addictive Behaviors* 37 (2012): 747–75.

76. Kerr et al., "Age-Period-Cohort Modelling"; Katherine M. Keyes and Richard Miech, "Age, Period, and Cohort Effects in Heavy Episodic Drinking in the US from 1985 to 2009," *Drug and Alcohol Dependence* 132 (2013): 140–48; Richard W. Wilsnack et al., "Are US Women Drinking Less (or More)? Historical and Aging Trends, 1981–2001," *Journal of Studies on Alcohol* 67 (2006): 341–48.

77. Breslow et al., "Trends in Alcohol Consumption Among Older Americans"; Grant et al., "Prevalence of 12-Month Alcohol Use"; Grucza et al., "Trends in Adult Alcohol Use."

78. Sharon C. Wilsnack and Richard W. Wilsnack, "Epidemiology of Women's Drinking," *Journal of Substance Abuse* 3 (1991): 133–57.

79. Knepper, "Women and the Impact of Addiction."

80. Norma Finkelstein, "Treatment Issues for Alcohol- and Drug-Dependent Pregnant and Parenting Women," *Health & Social Work* 19 (1994): 7–15.

81. Betty Friedan, *The Feminine Mystique* (New York: Dell Publishing, 1963).

82. Erick Trickey, "Inside the Story of America's 19th-Century Opiate Addiction," accessed June 10, 2021, https://www.smithsonianmag.com/history/inside-story-amer icas-19th-century-opiate-addiction-180967673/.

83. Sharon Druckerman and Sean Dooley, "Secret Life: Mom Confesses to Alcoholism," accessed July 9, 2018, https://abcnews.go.com/2020/mom-stress-mother hood-drove-drink/story?id=10488897.

84. Daniel M. Blonigen et al., "Socio-Contextual Factors Are Linked to Differences in the Course of Problem Drinking in Midlife: A Discordant-Twin Study," *The American Journal on Addictions* 24 (2015): 193–96; Kenneth E. Leonard and Rina D. Eiden, "Marital and Family Processes in the Context of Alcohol Use and Alcohol Disorders," *Annual Review of Clinical Psychology* 3 (2007): 285–310; Corrine Reczek et al., "Marital Histories and Heavy Alcohol Use Among Older Adults," *Journal of Health and Social Behavior* 57 (2016): 77–96.

85. Glen H. Elder, Monica Kirkpatrick Johnson, and Robert Crosnoe, "The Emergence and Development of Life Course Theory," in *Handbook of the Life Course*, ed. J. K. Mortimer and M. J. Shanahan (Boston, MA: Springer, 2003), 3–19.

86. Norella M. Putney and Vern L. Bengtson, "Intergenerational Relations in Changing Times," in *Handbook of the Life Course*, ed. J. K. Mortimer and M. J. Shanahan (Boston, MA: Springer, 2003), 149–64.

87. Karen G. Chartier, Nathaniel S. Thomas, and Kenneth S. Kendler, "Interrelationship Between Family History of Alcoholism and Generational Status in the Prediction of Alcohol Dependence in US Hispanics," *Psychological Medicine* 47 (2017): 137–47; Bridget F. Grant, Frederick S. Stinson, and Thomas C. Harford, "Age at Onset of Alcohol Use and DSM-IV Alcohol Abuse and Dependence: A 12-Year Follow-Up," *Journal of Substance Abuse* 13 (2001): 493–504; Kendler et al. "Transmission of Alcohol Use Disorder"; Muthén and Muthén, "The Development of Heavy Drinking."

88. Urie Brofenbrenner, "Ecological Systems Theory," in *International Encyclopedia of Psychology, Vol. 3*, ed. Alan E. Kazdin (Washington, DC: American Psychological Association, 2000), 129–33.

89. Allison M. Steiner and Paula C. Fletcher, "Sandwich Generation Caregiving: A Complex and Dynamic Role," *Journal of Adult Development* 24 (2017): 133–43.

90. Stephanie Boraas, "Volunteerism in the United States," *Monthly Labor Review* 126 (2003): 3; Peggy Petrzelka and Susan E. Mannon, "Keepin' This Little Town Going: Gender and Volunteerism in Rural America," *Gender & Society* 20 (2006): 236–58.

91. Reuben Hill, *Families Under Stress* (New York: Harper & Row, 1949).

92. Pauline Boss, "Family Stress," in *Handbook of Marriage and the Family*, ed. Marvin B Sussman and Suzanne K. Steinmetz (New York: Plenum Press, 1987); Hamilton I. McCubbin et al., "Family Stress and Coping: A Decade Review," *Journal of Marriage and the Family* 42 (1980): 855–71.

93. Haydon et al., "Beliefs Underlying Women's Intentions."

94. A. W. Geiger, Gretchen Livingston, and Kristen Bialik, "6 Facts About U.S. Moms," accessed June 12, 2021, https://www.pewresearch.org/fact-tank/2019/05/08

/facts-about-u-s-mothers/; U.S. Bureau of Labor Statistics, "Highlights of Women's Earnings in 2019," accessed June 12, 2021, https://www.bls.gov/opub/reports/womens-earnings/2019/pdf/home.pdf.

95. Frone, "Work Stress and Alcohol Use."

96. Tammy D. Allen et al., "Consequences Associated with Work-to-family Conflict: A Review and Agenda for Future Research," *Journal of Occupational Health Psychology* 5 (2000): 278–308; Rosalind C. Barnett and Grace K. Baruch, "Women's Involvement in Multiple Roles and Psychological Distress," *Journal of Personality and Social Psychology* 49 (1985): 135–45; Sheldon Cohen and Denise Janicki-Deverts, "Who's Stressed? Distributions of Psychological Stress in the United States in Probability Samples from 1983, 2006, and 2009," *Journal of Applied Social Psychology* 42 (2012): 1320–34; Susan Nolen-Hoeksema, "Gender Differences in Depression," *Current Directions in Psychological Science* 10 (2001): 173–76; Debra Umberson, Tetyana Pudrovska, and Corinne Reczek, "Parenthood, Childlessness, and Well-Being: A Life Course Perspective," *Journal of Marriage and Family* 72 (2010): 612–29; Frone, "Relationship of Work-Family Conflict to Substance Use"; Grzywacz and Marks, "Family, Work, Work-Family Spillover."

97. NIAAA, "Recommended Alcohol Questions," accessed July 10, 2020, https://www.niaaa.nih.gov/research/guidelines-and-resources/recommended-alcohol-questions.

98. NIAAA, "Alcohol Use Disorder: A Comparison Between DSM-IV and DSM-5," accessed July 7, 2020, https://www.niaaa.nih.gov/publications/brochures-and-fact-sheets/alcohol-use-disorder-comparison-between-dsm.

99. Lisa Bowleg, "When Black + Lesbian + Woman ≠ Black Lesbian Woman: The Methodological Challenges of Qualitative and Quantitative Intersectionality Research," *Sex Roles* 59 (2008): 312–25; Quora, "What Is the Intersection Theory in Sociology?" accessed June 12, 2021, https://www.quora.com/What-is-the-intersection-theory-in-sociology.

100. National Institute on Drug Abuse, "Monitoring the Future," accessed June 12, 2021, https://www.drugabuse.gov/drug-topics/trends-statistics/infographics/monitoring-future-2019-survey-results-overall-findings.

CHAPTER TWO

1. Elizabeth Hanford Dole et al., *Alcohol in America: Taking Action to Prevent Abuse* (Washington, D.C.: National Academies Press, 1985), 1.

2. Dole, *Alcohol in America.*

3. Gallup, "Alcohol and Drinking."

4. Matthew R. Pearson, Megan Kirouac, and Katie Witkiewitz, "Questioning the Validity of the 4+/5+ Binge or Heavy Drinking Criterion in College and Clinical Populations," *Addiction* 111 (2016): 1720–26.

5. Kerr et al., "Health Risk Factors Associated with Lifetime Abstinence from Alcohol."

6. Sarah A. Benton, "Social Drinkers, Problem Drinkers, and Alcoholics," accessed June 13, 2021, https://www.psychologytoday.com/us/blog/the-high-function ing-alcoholic/200904/social-drinkers-problem-drinkers-and-alcoholics.

7. Mintel Press Office, "Alcohol Manufacturers Drink in Profits from At-Home Consumption, Reports Mintel," accessed January 15, 2020, https://www.mintel .com/press-centre/food-and-drink/alcohol-manufacturers-drink-in-profits-from-at -home-consumption-reports-mintel#:~:text=Among%20alcohol%20drinkers %2C%2090%25%20consume,5.7.

8. U.S. Census Bureau, "U.S. Census Bureau Releases 2018 Families and Living Arrangements Tables," accessed January 15, 2021, https://www.census.gov/newsroom /press-releases/2018/families.html; U.S. Census Bureau, "America's Families and Living Arrangements: 2019," accessed January 15, 2021, https://www.census.gov/data /tables/2019/demo/families/cps-2019.html.

9. USDA, "Dietary Guidelines for Americans, 2020–2025," accessed April 21, 2021, https://www.dietaryguidelines.gov/sites/default/files/2021-03/Dietary_Guide lines_for_Americans-2020-2025.pdf.

10. Esser et al., "Peer Reviewed: Prevalence of Alcohol Dependence."

CHAPTER THREE

1. Jo Cranwell, Magdalena Opazo-Breton, and John Britton, "Adult and Adolescent Exposure to Tobacco and Alcohol Content in Contemporary YouTube Music Videos in Great Britain: A Population Estimate," *Journal of Epidemiology and Community Health* 70 (2016): 488–92; OECD, *Tackling Harmful Alcohol Use.*

2. Brenda L. Curtis et al., "Meta-Analysis of the Association of Alcohol-Related Social Media Use with Alcohol Consumption and Alcohol-Related Problems in Adolescents and Young Adults," *Alcoholism: Clinical and Experimental Research* 42 (2018): 978–86; David Jernigan et al., "Alcohol Marketing and Youth Alcohol Consumption: A Systematic Review of Longitudinal Studies Published Since 2008," *Addiction* 112 (2017): 7–20; Megan A. Moreno et al., "Testing Young Adults' Reactions to Facebook Cues and Their Associations with Alcohol Use," *Substance Use and Misuse* 54 (2019): 1450–460.

3. Alvarez, Brenda, "All Hands on Deck: School-Based Programs to Stem Substance Use," accessed January 16, 2021, https://www.nea.org/advocating-for-change /new-from-nea/all-hands-deck-school-based-programs-stem-substance-abuse; Drug Policy Alliance, "Real Drug Education," accessed January 16, 2021, https://drug policy.org/issues/real-drug-education.

4. Katelyn Newman, "A Different Dose of Drug Education," accessed January 16, 2021, https://www.usnews.com/news/healthiest-communities/articles/2019-11-14 /high-school-drug-curriculum-includes-harm-reduction-emphasis.

5. Sandra C. Jones and Chloe S. Gordon, "A Systematic Review of Children's Alcohol-Related Knowledge, Attitudes and Expectancies," *Preventive Medicine* 105 (2017): 19–31.

6. Lloyd D. Johnston et al., *Monitoring the Future National Survey Results on Drug Use, 1975–2017: Overview, Key Findings on Adolescent Drug Use* (Ann Arbor, MI: Institute for Social Research, the University of Michigan, 2018).

7. Casey Bohrman et al., "Being Superwoman: Low Income Mothers Surviving Problem Drinking and Intimate Partner Violence," *Journal of Family Violence* 32 (2017): 699–709, 704.

8. Jones and Gordon, "A Systematic Review"; Donald A. Brand et al., "Comparative Analysis of Alcohol Control Policies in 30 Countries," *PLoS Medicine* 4 (2007): e15; Won Kim Cook, Jason Bond, and Thomas K. Greenfield, "Are Alcohol Policies Associated with Alcohol Consumption in Low- and Middle-Income Countries?" *Addiction* 109 (2014): 1081–90.

9. David J. DeWit et al., "Age at First Alcohol Use: A Risk Factor for the Development of Alcohol Disorders," *American Journal of Psychiatry* 157 (2000): 745–50; Carolyn E. Sartor et al., "Timing of First Alcohol Use and Alcohol Dependence: Evidence of Common Genetic Influences," *Addiction* 104 (2009): 1512–18; Wing See Yuen et al., "Adolescent Alcohol Use Trajectories: Risk Factors and Adult Outcomes," *Pediatrics* 146 (2020), doi: 10.1542/peds.2020-0440.

10. Emmanuel Kuntsche, "'Do Grown-Ups Become Happy When They Drink?' Alcohol Expectancies Among Preschoolers," *Experimental and Clinical Psychopharmacology* 25 (2017): 24.

11. Megan Cook, Koen Smit, Carmen Voogt, and Emmanuel Kuntsche, "Alcohol-Related Cognitions Among Children Aged 2–12: Where Do They Originate from and How Do They Develop?" in R. Cooke, D. Conroy, E. L. Davies, M. S. Hagger, and R. O. de Visser (eds.) *The Palgrave Handbook of Psychological Perspectives on Alcohol Consumption* (London: Palgrave Macmillan, 2021), 351.

12. Judy A. Andrews and Missy Peterson, "The Development of Social Images of Substance Users in Children: A Guttman Unidimensional Scaling Approach," *Journal of Substance Use* 11 (2006): 305–21.

13. Jones and Gordon, "A Systematic Review."

14. Koen Smit et al., "Exposure to Parental Alcohol Use Rather Than Parental Drinking Shapes Offspring's Alcohol Expectancies," *Alcoholism: Clinical and Experimental Research* 43 (2019): 1967–77.

15. Brand et al., "Comparative Analysis of Alcohol Control Policies"; Cook et al., "Are Alcohol Policies Associated with Alcohol Consumption?"

16. GBD 2016 Alcohol Collaborators, "Alcohol Use and Burden for 195 Countries and Territories."

17. Sonia Sharmin et al., "Effects of Parental Alcohol Rules on Risky Drinking and Related Problems in Adolescence: Systematic Review and Meta-Analysis," *Drug and Alcohol Dependence* 178 (2017): 243–56.

18. Amy Schalet, *Not Under My Roof: Parents, Teens, and the Culture of Sex* (Chicago, IL: University of Chicago Press, 2011).

19. Schalet, *Not Under My Roof*, 82.

20. Jeremy Berke, Shayanne Gal, and Yeji Jesse Lee, "Marijuana Legalization Is Sweeping the US: See Every State Where Cannabis Is Legal," accessed May 24, 2021, https://www.businessinsider.com/legal-marijuana-states-2018-1.

21. Megan Brenan, "Support for Legal Marijuana Inches Up to a New High of 68%," accessed January 19, 2021, https://news.gallup.com/poll/323582/support -legal-marijuana-inches-new-high.aspx; Jeffrey M. Jones, "Most in U.S. Say Consuming Alcohol, Marijuana Morally OK," accessed January 19, 2021, https://news .gallup.com/poll/235250/say-consuming-alcohol-marijuana-morally.aspx.

22. Zach Hrynowski, "What Percentage of Americans Smoke Marijuana?" accessed January 18, 2021, https://news.gallup.com/poll/284135/percentage-americans-smoke -marijuana.aspx.

23. Alyssa Davis, "In U.S., Opioids Viewed as Most Serious Local Drug Problem," accessed January 19, 2021, https://news.gallup.com/poll/194042/opioids -viewed-serious-local-drug-problem.aspx.

24. History.com, "War on Drugs," accessed May 5, 2021, https://www.history.com /topics/crime/the-war-on-drugs#section_5.

CHAPTER FOUR

1. Fingarette, *Heavy Drinking*, 16.

2. Fingarette, *Heavy Drinking*, 17.

3. Robert Ezra Park and Ernest Watson Burgess. *Introduction to the Science of Sociology* (Glasgow, Scotland: Good Press, 2019).

4. Mira Mayrhofer and Jörg Matthes, "Drinking at Work: The Portrayal of Alcohol in Workplace-Related TV Dramas," *Mass Communication and Society* 21 (2018): 94–114, 95.

5. Curtis et al., "Meta-Analysis of the Association of Alcohol-Related Social Media Use"; Jernigan et al., "Alcohol Marketing and Youth Alcohol Consumption"; Moreno et al., "Testing Young Adults' Reactions to Facebook Cues."

6. Waseem Akram and Rekesh Kumar, "A Study on Positive and Negative Effects of Social Media on Society," *International Journal of Computer Sciences and Engineering* 5 (2017): 351–54; Donna Freitas, *The Happiness Effect: How Social Media Is Driving a Generation to Appear Perfect at Any Cost* (Oxford, England: Oxford University Press, 2017); Su-Jung Nam, "Mediating Effect of Social Support on the Relationship Between Older Adults' Use of Social Media and Their Quality-of-Life," *Current Psychology* (2019): 1–9; Jacqueline W. Nesi et al., "Friends' Alcohol-Related Social Networking Site Activity Predicts Escalations in Adolescent Drinking: Mediation by Peer Norms," *Journal of Adolescent Health* 60 (2017): 641–47.

7. Curtis et al., "Meta-Analysis of the Association of Alcohol-Related Social Media Use."

8. Moreno et al., "Testing Young Adults' Reactions to Facebook Cues"; Megan A. Moreno and Jennifer M. Whitehill, "Influence of Social Media on Alcohol Use in Adolescents and Young Adults," *Alcohol Research: Current Reviews* 36 (2014): 91.

9. Erving Goffman, *The Presentation of Self in Everyday Life* (Garden City, NY: Doubleday Anchor Books, 1959).

10. Anne Werner and Kirsti Malterud, "Children of Parents with Alcohol Problems Performing Normality: A Qualitative Interview Study About Unmet Needs for

Professional Support," *International Journal of Qualitative Studies on Health and Well-Being* 11 (2016): 1–11, 6.

11. Emily Nicholls, *Negotiating Femininities in the Neoliberal Night-Time Economy: Too Much of a Girl?* (Cham, Switzerland: Springer, 2018), 89.

12. Christopher Cheers, Sarah Callinan, and Amy Pennay, "The 'Sober Eye': Examining Attitudes Towards Non-Drinkers in Australia," *Psychology and Health* 36 (2020): 385–404.

13. Dann, *The Wine O'Clock Myth,* 25–26.

14. Dann, *The Wine O'Clock Myth,* 159.

15. Rocco L. Capraro, "Why College Men Drink: Alcohol, Adventure, and the Paradox of Masculinity," *Journal of American College Health* 48 (2000): 307–15.

16. Hope Landrine, Stephen Bardwell, and Tina Dean, "Gender Expectations for Alcohol Use: A Study of the Significance of the Masculine Role," *Sex Roles* 19 (1988): 703–12.

17. Abbey and Harnish, "Perception of Sexual Intent"; Gomberg, "Women and Alcoholism"; Lyons and Willott, "Alcohol Consumption"; Ricciardelli et al., "Marital Histories."

18. Abigail R. Riemer et al., "She Looks Like She'd Be an Animal in Bed: Dehumanization of Drinking Women in Social Contexts," *Sex Roles* 80 (2019): 617–29.

19. Cheers et al., "The Sober Eye," 11.

20. Nicolls, *Negotiating Femininities.* Fiona Measham, "'Doing Gender'—'Doing Drugs': Conceptualizing the Gendering of Drug Cultures," *Contemporary Drug Problems* 29 (2002): 335–73, 363.

21. Measham, "Doing Gender," 146.

22. Wilsnack et al., "Are US Women Drinking Less (or More)"; Richard W. Wilsnack, Sharon C. Wilsnack, and Isidore S. Obot, "Why Study Gender, Alcohol and Culture?" in *Alcohol, Gender and Drinking Problems: Perspectives from Low and Middle Income Countries* (Geneva, Switzerland: World Health Organization, 2005), 1–25.

23. Laura F. Kleinand and Lillian A. Ackerman, *Women and Power in Native North America* (Norman, OK: University of Oklahoma Press, 1995).

24. Karen Chartier and Raul Caetano, "Ethnicity and Health Disparities in Alcohol Research," *Alcohol Research & Health* 33 (2010): 152–60.

25. Karen Codazzi, Valéria Pero, and André Albuquerque Sant'Anna, "Social Norms and Female Labor Participation in Brazil," *Review of Development Economics* 22 (2018): 1513–35; Florence Kerr-Corrêa et al., "Differences in Drinking Patterns Between Men and Women in Brazil," in *Alcohol, Gender and Drinking Problems,* ed. Isidore S. Obat and Robin Room (Geneva, Switzerland: World Health Organization, 2005), 49–68.

26. Nicholls, "Negotiating Femininities," 8.

27. Christine Griffin, "Good Girls, Bad Girls: Anglocentrism and Diversity in the Constitution of Contemporary Girlhood," in *All About the Girl: Culture, Power, and Identity,* ed. Anita Harris (New York: Routledge, 2004), 29–43; Anita Harris, "Jamming Girl Culture: Young Women and Consumer Citizenship," in *All About the Girl: Culture, Power, and Identity,* ed. Anita Harris (New York: Routledge, 2004), 163–72;

Mary Jane Kehily, "Taking Centre Stage? Girlhood and the Contradictions of Femininity Across Three Generations," *Girlhood Studies* 1 (2008): 51–71.

28. Dawn Currie, Deirdre M. Kelly, and Shauna Pomerantz, *"Girl Power": Girls Reinventing Girlhood*, Vol. 4 (New York: Peter Lang, 2009).

29. Lisa Wade and Myra Marx Ferree, *Gender: Ideas, Interactions, and Institutions* (New York: W. W. Norton, 2019), 164.

30. Ben Milne, "How Babycham Changed British Drinking Habits," accessed January 31, 2021, https://www.bbc.com/news/magazine-25302633.

31. Philip Norman, *Babycham Night* (London: Pan Publishing, 2011), xii.

32. Esser et al., "Peer Reviewed: Prevalence of Alcohol Dependence"; Jones, "Drinking Highest Among Educated Upper-Income Americans"; Keating, "Nine Charts That Show How White Women Are Drinking Themselves to Death."

33. Mayrhofer and Matthes, "Drinking at Work."

34. Michael R. Frone, "Prevalence and Distribution of Alcohol Use and Impairment in the Workplace: A US National Survey," *Journal of Studies on Alcohol* 67 (2006): 147–56.

35. Jack K. Martin, Joan M. Kraft, and Paul M. Roman, "Extent and Impact of Alcohol and Drug Use Problems in the Workplace," in *Drug Testing in the Workplace*, ed. Scott Macdonald and Paul Roman (Boston, MA: Springer, 1994), 3–31; Susan K. McFarlin and William Fals-Stewart, "Workplace Absenteeism and Alcohol Use: A Sequential Analysis," *Psychology of Addictive Behaviors* 16 (2002): 17.

36. Kristin Buvik, "It's Time for a Drink! Alcohol as an Investment in the Work Environment," *Drugs: Education, Prevention and Policy* 27 (2020): 86–91.

37. Frone, "Work Stress and Alcohol Use."

38. Jersild, *Happy Hours*, 132

39. Genevieve M. Ames and Joel W. Grube, "Alcohol Availability and Workplace Drinking: Mixed Method Analyses," *Journal of Studies on Alcohol* 60 (1999): 383–93.

CHAPTER FIVE

1. Caetano et al., "The Epidemiology of Drinking"; Cho and Crittenden, "The Impact of Adult Roles"; Grant et al., "Epidemiology of DSM-5 Alcohol Use Disorder"; Johnson et al., "Drinking Over the Life Course"; Laborde and Mair, "Alcohol Use Patterns Among Postpartum Women."

2. Sarah McKetta and Katherine M. Keyes, "Heavy and Binge Alcohol Drinking and Parenting Status in the United States from 2006 to 2018: An Analysis of Nationally Representative Cross-Sectional Surveys," *PLoS Medicine* 16 (2019): e1002954.

3. Janet Kay Bobo et al., "Predicting 10-year Alcohol Use Trajectories Among Men Age 50 Years and Older," *The American Journal of Geriatric Psychiatry* 21 (2013): 204–213; Breslow et al., "Trends in Alcohol Consumption Among Older Americans"; Grant et al., "Prevalence of 12-Month Alcohol Use"; Grucza et al., "Trends in Adult Alcohol Use"; Annie Britton et al., "Life Course Trajectories of

Alcohol Consumption in the United Kingdom Using Longitudinal Data from Nine Cohort Studies," *BMC Medicine* 13 (2015): 1–9.

4. Joan Curlee, "Alcoholism and the 'Empty Nest,'" *Bulletin of the Menninger Clinic* 33 (1969): 165–71; Gomberg, "Women and Alcoholism"; Edith S. Lisansky Gomberg, "Risk Factors for Drinking over a Woman's Life Span," *Alcohol Health and Research World* 18 (1994): 220; Richard W. Wilsnack and Randall Cheloha, "Women's Roles and Problem Drinking Across the Lifespan," *Social Problems* 34 (1987): 231–48; Woolf and Schoomaker, "Life Expectancy and Mortality Rates"; Stewart et al., "Mothers' Alcohol Use."

5. Breslow et al., "Trends in Alcohol Consumption"; Britton et al., "Life Course Trajectories"; Grucza et al., "Trends in Adult Alcohol Use."

6. Geiger et al., "Six Facts About U.S. Moms"; Sarah Jane Glynn, "Breadwinning Mothers Continue to Be the U.S. Norm," accessed June 21, 2020, https://www.ameri canprogress.org/issues/women/reports/2019/05/10/469739/breadwinning-mothers -continue-u-s-norm/; U.S. Bureau of Labor Statistics, "Highlights of Women's Earn- ings in 2019."

7. Jennifer L. Hook, "Women's Housework: New Tests of Time and Money," *Journal of Marriage and Family* 79 (2017): 179–98.

8. Gretchen Livingston and Kim Parker, "8 Facts About American Dads," accessed February 12, 2021, https://www.pewresearch.org/fact-tank/2019/06/12 /fathers-day-facts/.

9. Arlie Hochschild, *The Second Shift* (New York: Avon Books, 1989); David J. Maume, Rachel A. Sebastian, and Anthony R. Bardo, "Gender, Work-Family Re- sponsibilities, and Sleep," *Gender & Society* 24 (2010): 746–68; Susan Thistle, *From Marriage to the Market: The Transformation of Women's Lives and Work* (Berkeley, CA: University of California Press, 2006).

10. Claire M. Kamp Dush, Jill E. Yavorsky, and Sarah J. Schoppe-Sullivan, "What Are Men Doing While Women Perform Extra Unpaid Labor? Leisure and Specializa- tion at the Transitions to Parenthood," *Sex Roles* 78 (2018): 715–30; Joanna R. Pepin, Liana C. Sayer, and Lynne M. Casper, "Marital Status and Mothers' Time Use: Child- care, Housework, Leisure, and Sleep," *Demography* 55 (2018): 107–33.

11. Sarah Flood, Ann Meier, and Kelly Musick, "Reassessing Parents' Leisure Quality with Direct Measures of Well-Being: Do Children Detract from Parents' Down Time?" *Journal of Marriage and Family* 82 (2020): 1326–39; Liana C. Sayer, "Parenthood and Leisure Time Disparities," in *Contemporary Parenting and Parent- hood: From News Headlines to New Research*, ed. Michelle Y. Janning (Santa Bar- bara, CA: ABC-CLIO, 2018), 168–98.

12. U.S. Census Bureau, "U.S. Census Bureau Releases."

13. Timothy Grall, "Custodial Mothers and Fathers and Their Child Support: 2017," accessed February 12, 2020, https://www.census.gov/content/dam/Census /library/publications/2020/demo/p60-269.pdf.

14. Lisa F. Berkman and Thomas Glass, "Social Integration, Social Networks, Social Support, and Health," *Social Epidemiology* 1 (2000): 137–73; Lixia Ge et al., "Social Isolation, Loneliness and Their Relationships with Depressive Symptoms: A Population-Based Study," *PLoS One* 12 (2017): e0182145; Linda A. Liang, Ursula

Berger, and Christian Brand, "Psychosocial Factors Associated with Symptoms of Depression, Anxiety and Stress Among Single Mothers with Young Children: A Population-Based Study," *Journal of Affective Disorders* 242 (2019): 255–64; Emily J. Passias, Liana Sayer, and Joanna R. Pepin, "Who Experiences Leisure Deficits? Mothers' Marital Status and Leisure Time," *Journal of Marriage and Family* 79 (2017): 1001–22; Stephanie Schrempft et al., "Associations Between Social Isolation, Loneliness, and Objective Physical Activity in Older Men and Women," *BMC Public Health* 19 (2019): 1–10; Zoe E. Taylor and Rand D. Conger, "Promoting Strengths and Resilience in Single-Mother Families," *Child Development* 88 (2017): 350–55; Peggy A. Thoits, "Mechanisms Linking Social Ties and Support to Physical and Mental Health," *Journal of Health and Social Behavior* 52 (2011): 145–61.

15. Allen et al., "Consequences Associated with Work-to-family Conflict"; Barnett and Baruch, "Women's Involvement in Multiple Roles"; Kathleen T. Brady and Susan C. Sonne, "The Role of Stress in Alcohol Use, Alcoholism Treatment, and Relapse," *Alcohol Research & Health* 23 (1999): 263–71; Frone, "Work Stress and Alcohol Use"; Frone et al., "Relationship of Work-Family Conflict to Substance Use."

16. Grzywacz and Marks, "Family, Work, Work-Family Spillover."

17. Frone, Russell, and Cooper, "Relationship of Work-Family Conflict."

18. Frone, "Work Stress and Alcohol Use."

19. Geiger et al., "6 Facts About U.S. Moms."

20. Livingston and Parker, "8 Facts About American Dads."

21. Knepper, "Women and the Impact of Addiction."

22. Jennifer Brady et al., "A Systematic Review of the Salient Role of Feminine Norms on Substance Use Among Women," *Addictive Behaviors* 62 (2016): 83–90.

23. Sharon Hayes, *The Cultural Contradictions of Motherhood* (New Haven, CT: Yale University Press, 1996).

24. Sarah Cottrell, "How Mommy Drinking Culture Has Normalized Alcoholism for Women in America," accessed July 10, 2021, https://www.babble.com/parenting/mommy-drinking-culture-wine-motherhood/.

25. Claire Howorth, "Motherhood Is Hard to Get Wrong. So Why Do so Many Moms Feel so Bad About Themselves?" accessed July 10, 2021, http://time.com/magazine/us/4989032/october-30th-2017-vol-190-no-18-u-s/; Raine, *Women's Perspectives on Drugs and Alcohol.*

26. Betty Friedan, *The Feminine Mystique, 10th Anniversary Edition* (New York: Dell Publishing, 1974); Friedan's study was based on a sample of white women who had graduated with her from Smith College and does not capture the experiences of women with less education and lower incomes, and women of color.

27. Scary Mommy, "Scary Mommy Confessions: When You're a Mom Who Drinks," accessed February 20, 2021, https://www.scarymommy.com/mothering-drinking/.

28. Ben Killingsworth, "'Drinking Stories' from a Playgroup: Alcohol in the Lives of Middle-Class Mothers in Australia," *Ethnography* 7 (2006): 357–84, 372, 375.

29. Ashley Fetters, "The Many Faces of the 'Wine Mom,'" accessed February 13, 2021, https://www.theatlantic.com/family/archive/2020/05/wine-moms-explained/612001/.

30. Fetters, "The Many Faces of the 'Wine Mom.'"

31. Samantha Cassetty, "Pedialyte and Other Good Ways to Bounce Back from a Hangover," accessed July 10, 2021, https://www.nbcnews.com/better/pop-culture/best-way-bounce-back-hangover-ncna861326; Jeanette Settembre, "Pedialyte Is the Hottest Hangover Cure, but Does It Really Work?" accessed July 10, 2021, https://www.marketwatch.com/story/pedialyte-is-the-hottest-hangover-cure-but-does-it-really-work-2018-12-31; Kaitlyn Tiffany, "How Pedialyte Got Pedialit," accessed July 10, 2021, https://www.vox.com/the-goods/2018/9/10/17819358/pedialyte-hangover-marketing-strategy-instagram-influencers.

32. Julie Scagell, "Someone Invented Wine Juice Boxes Because We Deserve to Be Happy," accessed July 10, 2021, https://www.scarymommy.com/high-key-portable-wine-pouches/.

33. Raine, *Women's Perspectives on Drugs and Alcohol*.

34. Jo Littler, "Mothers Behaving Badly: Chaotic Hedonism and the Crisis of Neoliberal Social Reproduction," *Cultural Studies* 34 (2020): 499–520, 499.

35. Oxford English Dictionary, "Ladette," accessed February 15, 2021, https://www.lexico.com/en/definition/ladette.

36. Sarah Turner and Lucy Rocca, *The Sober Revolution: Women Calling Time on Wine O'Clock* (Abercynon, Wales: Accent Press Ltd., 2013), 10.

37. Emelda Whelehan, *Overloaded: Popular Culture and the Future of Feminism* (London, England: The Women's Press, 2000), 9.

38. Raine, *Women's Perspectives on Drugs and Alcohol*, 37.

39. Cydney Henderson, "Chrissy Teigen Explains Why She Quit Drinking, Praises Book That Inspired Lifestyle Change," accessed February 13, 2021, https://www.usatoday.com/story/entertainment/celebrities/2020/12/31/chrissy-teigen-reveals-shes-4-weeks-sober-why-she-quit-drinking/4097801001/.

40. Harper's Bazaar, "Anne Hathaway on Giving Up Alcohol: 'It's Irritating How Well It's Going," accessed February 13, 2021, https://www.harpersbazaar.com/uk/celebrities/news/a27249916/anne-hathaway-giving-up-alcohol/.

41. Julie Ward Dereshinsky, "The Uneventful Monday Night That Made Me Stop Drinking," accessed February 20, 2021, https://www.scarymommy.com/uneventful-monday-night-stop-drinking/.

42. Bohrman et al., "Being Superwoman," 704.

43. Ashley Abramson, "The Cheeky 'Wine Mom' Trope Isn't Just Dumb. It's Dangerous," accessed February 13, 2021, http:/www.washingtonpost.com/news/parenting/wp/2018/09/21/the-cheeky-wine-mom-trope-isnt-just-dumb-its-dangerous/.

44. Nicole Pelletiere, "'A Pump-and-Dump Kind of Day': How Wine-Mom Culture Shifted from Funny Memes to Unhappy Hangovers" accessed February 13, 2021, https://www.goodmorningamerica.com/family/story/pump-dump-kind-day-wine-mom-culture-shifted-62625309.

45. Martha Carucci, *Sobrietease* (Alexandria, VA: Sobrietease, 2016).

CHAPTER SIX

1. Leonard and Eiden, "Marital and Family Processes," 285.

2. Diane N. Lye, "Adult Child–Parent Relationships," *Annual Review of Sociology* 22 (1996): 79–102.

3. Bohrman et al., "Being Superwoman," 705–706.

4. Jane Ribbens McCarthy, Val Gillies, and Carol-Ann Hooper, "'Family Troubles' and 'Troubling Families': Opening Up Fertile Ground," *Journal of Family Issues* 40 (2019): 2207–24.

5. Lucy Blake, "Parents and Children Who Are Estranged in Adulthood: A Review and Discussion of the Literature," *Journal of Family Theory & Review* 9 (2017): 521–36.

6. Boss, "Family Stress."

7. Kylie Agllias, "Family Estrangement: Aberration or Common Occurrence?" accessed July 11, 2021, https://www.psychologytoday.com/us/blog/family-conflict/201409/family-estrangement-aberration-or-common-occurrence-0; Kylie Agllias, "Family Estrangement," in *Encyclopedia of Social Work*, ed. Cynthia Franklin (Oxford, England: National Association of Social Workers Press and Oxford University Press, 2013); Kylie Agllias, *Family Estrangement: A Matter of Perspective* (Oxon: Routledge, 2017).

8. Blake, "Parents and Children Who Are Estranged"; Kristina M. Scharp and Elizabeth Dorrance Hall, "Family Marginalization, Alienation, and Estrangement: Questioning the Nonvoluntary Status of Family Relationships," *Annals of the International Communication Association* 41 (2017): 28–45.

9. Richard P. Conti, "Family Estrangement: Establishing a Prevalence Rate," *Journal of Psychology and Behavioral Science* 3 (2015): 28–35; Jennifer Davis-Berman, "Older Men in the Homeless Shelter: In-Depth Conversations Lead to Practice Implications," *Journal of Gerontological Social Work* 54 (2011): 456–74.

10. Agglias, *Family Estrangement*; Audrey Linden and Elizabeth Sillence, "'I'm Finally Allowed to Be Me': Parent-Child Estrangement and Psychological Wellbeing," *Families, Relationships and Societies* 10, no. 2 (2021): 325–41. doi: 10.1332/204674319x15647593365505.

11. Russell A. Ward, Glenna Spitze, and Glenn Deane, "The More the Merrier? Multiple Parent–Adult Child Relations," *Journal of Marriage and Family* 71 (2009): 161–73.

12. Rosemary Blieszner and Karen A. Roberto, "Friendship Across the Life Span: Reciprocity in Individual and Relationship Development," in *Growing Together: Personal Relationships Across the Life Span*, ed. Frieder R. Lang and Karen L. Fingerman (Cambridge, NY: Cambridge University Press, 2004), 159–82; Masako Ishii-Kuntz, "Social Interaction and Psychological Well-Being: Comparison Across Stages of Adulthood," *The International Journal of Aging and Human Development* 30 (1990): 15–36.

13. Simone de Beauvoir, *The Second Sex* (New York: Vintage, 1989); Mary Lee A. Roberts and Martin Schiavenato, "Othering in the Nursing Context: A Concept Analysis," *Nursing Open* 4 (2017): 174–81, 174.

14. Sophia E. Chambers et al., "Alcohol Use and Breast Cancer Risk: A Qualitative Study of Women's Perspectives to Inform the Development of a Preventative Intervention in Breast Clinics," *European Journal of Cancer Care* 28 (2019): e13075.

15. Gretchen Livingston, "More Than One-in-Ten U.S. Parents Are Also Caring for an Adult," accessed February 12, 2021, https://www.pewresearch.org/fact-tank /2018/11/29/more-than-one-in-ten-u-s-parents-are-also-caring-for-an-adult.

16. Anne Shaffer and Byron Egeland, "Intergenerational Transmission of Familial Boundary Dissolution: Observations and Psychosocial Outcomes in Adolescence," *Family Relations* 60 (2011): 290–302.

17. Leonard and Eiden, "Marital and Family Processes," 285.

18. Raine, *Women's Perspectives on Drugs and Alcohol*; Lorraine Smith, "Invited Review: Help Seeking in Alcohol-Dependent Females," *Alcohol and Alcoholism* 27 (1992): 3–9.

CHAPTER SEVEN

1. Holly Whitaker, "The Patriarchy of Alcoholics Anonymous," accessed July 11, 2021, https://www.nytimes.com/2019/12/27/opinion/alcoholics-anonymous-women .html.

2. Nicolls, *Negotiating Femininities*.

3. Jenna Hollenstein, *Drinking to Distraction* (Morrisville, NC: Lulu Publishing, 2014).

4. Turner and Rocca, *The Sober Revolution*, 6–7.

5. Jonathan Henssler, Martin Müller, Helena Carreira, Tom Bschor, Andreas Heinz, and Christopher Baethge, "Controlled Drinking—Non-abstinent versus Abstinent Treatment Goals in Alcohol Use Disorder: A Systematic Review, Meta-analysis and Meta-regression." *Addiction* 116, no. 8 (2021): 1973–87.

6. Turner and Rocca, *The Sober Revolution*, 13 (italics added).

7. Lynn Stuart Parramore, "'Promising Young Woman'": Covid and the Women Giving Up Alcohol to Fight the Patriarchy," accessed July 11, 2021 (https://www .nbcnews.com/think/opinion/promising-young-woman-covid-women-giving-alcohol -fight-patriarchy-ncna1256229).

8. Philip J. Cook, *Paying the Tab: The Costs and Benefits of Alcohol Control* (Princeton, NJ: Princeton University Press, 2007).

9. Dann, *The Wine O'Clock Myth*.

10. Jersild, *Happy Hours*, 152.

11. Xiaoxin I. Yao et al., "Change in Moderate Alcohol Consumption and Quality of Life: Evidence from 2 Population-Based Cohorts," *CMAJ* 191 (2019): E753–60.

APPENDIX TABLE 1

1. Categories are not mutually exclusive and equal the total number of children of any age of the participants (N=41).

APPENDIX TABLE 2

1. "Immediate family" includes parents, children, siblings, spouses, and partners. "Extended family" includes other family members such as grandparents, aunts, uncles, cousins, etc.

2. The DSM-5 uses 11 criteria during the same 12-month period to diagnose the presence of an AUD (see Table 3). The presence of 2 to 3 symptoms is considered "mild," 4 to 5 symptoms is considered "moderate," and 6 or more symptoms is considered "severe."

Bibliography

Abbey, Antonia, and Richard J. Harnish. "Perception of Sexual Intent: The Role of Gender, Alcohol Consumption, and Rape Supportive Attitudes." *Sex Roles* 32 (1995): 297–313.

Abramson, Ashley. "The Cheeky 'Wine Mom' Trope Isn't Just Dumb. It's Dangerous." September 21, 2018, http:/www.washingtonpost.com/news/parenting/wp/2018/09/21/the-cheeky-wine-mom-trope-isnt-just-dumb-its-dangerous.

Acciai, Francesco, and Glenn Firebaugh. "Why Did Life Expectancy Decline in the United States in 2015? A Gender-Specific Analysis." *Social Science & Medicine* 190 (2017): 174–80.

Achenbach, Joel, and Dan Keating. "A New Divide in American Death." April 10, 2016, https://www.washingtonpost.com/sf/national/2016/04/10/a-new-divide-in-american-death/?tid=usw_passupdatepg.

Agllias, Kylie. "Family Estrangement: Aberration or Common Occurrence?" September 8, 2014, https://www.psychologytoday.com/us/blog/family-conflict/201409/family-estrangement-aberration-or-common-occurrence-0.

Agllias, Kylie. *Family Estrangement: A Matter of Perspective*. Oxon, UK: Routledge, 2017.

Akram, Waseem, and Rekesh Kumar. "A Study on Positive and Negative Effects of Social Media on Society." *International Journal of Computer Sciences and Engineering* 5 (2017): 351–54.

Allen, Tammy D., David E. L. Herst, Carly S. Bruck, and Martha Sutton. "Consequences Associated with Work-to-Family Conflict: A Review and Agenda for Future Research." *Journal of Occupational Health Psychology* 5 (2000): 278.

Alpers, Silvia Eiken, Jens Christoffer Skogen, Silje Mæland, Ståle Pallesen, Åsgeir Kjetland Rabben, Linn-Heidi Lunde, and Lars Thore Fadnes. "Alcohol Consumption During a Pandemic Lockdown Period and Change in Alcohol Consumption Related to Worries and Pandemic Measures." *International Journal of Environmental Research and Public Health* 18 (2021): 1220.

Alvarez, Brenda. "All Hands on Deck: School-Based Programs to Stem Substance Use." March 12, 2018, https://www.nea.org/advocating-for-change/new-from-nea /all-hands-deck-school-based-programs-stem-substance-abuse.

Amy, Schalet. *Not Under My Roof: Parents, Teens, and the Culture of Sex*. Chicago, IL: University of Chicago Press, 2011.

Andrews, Judy A., and Missy Peterson. "The Development of Social Images of Substance Users in Children: A Guttman Unidimensional Scaling Approach." *Journal of Substance Use* 11 (2006): 305–21.

Aubrey, Allison. "With Heavy Drinking on the Rise, How Much Is Too Much?" 16 Aug. 2017, http://www.npr.org/sections/thesalt/2017/08/16/543965637/women -who-love-wine-are-you-binge-drinking-without-realizing-it.

Avery, Ally R., Siny Tsang, Edmund Y. W. Seto, and Glen E. Duncan. "Stress, Anxiety, and Change in Alcohol Use During the COVID-19 Pandemic: Findings Among Adult Twin Pairs." *Frontiers in Psychiatry* 11 (2020), doi: 10.3389 /fpsyt.2020.571084.

Balan, Sundari, Gregory Widner, Hsing-Jung Chen, Darrell Hudson, Sarah Gehlert, and Rumi Kato Price. "Motherhood, Psychological Risks, and Resources in Relation to Alcohol Use Disorder: Are There Differences Between Black and White Women?" *International Scholarly Research Notices* (2014), doi: 10.1155/2014/437080.

Barnett, Rosalind C., and Grace K. Baruch. "Women's Involvement in Multiple Roles and Psychological Distress." *Journal of Personality and Social Psychology* 49 (1985): 135–45.

Benton, Sarah A. "Caron Study Reveals 'Top 5 Reasons' Mothers Turn to Alcohol." May 10, 2013, https://www.psychologytoday.com/blog/the-high-functioning-alco holic/201305/caron-study-reveals-top-5-reasons-mothers-turn-alcohol.

Benton, Sarah A. "Social Drinkers, Problem Drinkers, and Alcoholics," April 28, 2009, https://www.psychologytoday.com/us/blog/the-high-functioning-alcoholic /200904/social-drinkers-problem-drinkers-and-alcoholics.

Berke, Jeremy, Shayanne Gal, and Yeji Jesse Lee. "Marijuana Legalization Is Sweeping the US: See Every State Where Cannabis Is Legal." July 9, 2021, https://www .businessinsider.com/legal-marijuana-states-2018-1.

Berkman, Lisa F., and Thomas Glass. "Social Integration, Social Networks, Social Support, and Health." *Social Epidemiology* 1 (2000): 137–73.

Biddle, Nicholas, Ben Edwards, Matthew Gray, and Kate Sollis. "Alcohol Consumption During the COVID-19 Period: May 2020." June 10, 2020, https:// openresearch-repository.anu.edu.au/bitstream/1885/213196/1/Alcohol_consump tion_during_the_COVID-19_period.pdf.

Blieszner, Rosemary, and Karen A. Roberto. "Friendship Across the Life Span: Reciprocity in Individual and Relationship Development." in *Growing Together: Personal Relationships Across the Life Span*, edited by Frieder R. Lang and Karen L. Fingerman, 159–82. Cambridge, NY: Cambridge University Press, 2004.

Blonigen, Daniel M., Thomas Burroughs, Jon Randolph Haber, and Theodore Jacob. "Socio-Contextual Factors Are Linked to Differences in the Course of Problem Drinking in Midlife: A Discordant-Twin Study." *The American Journal on Addictions* 24 (2015): 193–96.

Bobo, Janet Kay, April A. Greek, Daniel H. Klepinger, and Jerald R. Herting. "Predicting 10-Year Alcohol Use Trajectories Among Men Age 50 Years and Older." *The American Journal of Geriatric Psychiatry* 21 (2013): 204–13.

Boden, Joseph M., and David M. Fergusson. "Alcohol and Depression." *Addiction* 106 (2011): 906–14.

Bohrman, Casey, Julie Tennille, Kimberly Levin, Melissa Rodgers, and Karin Rhodes. "Being Superwoman: Low Income Mothers Surviving Problem Drinking and Intimate Partner Violence." *Journal of Family Violence* 32 (2017): 699–709.

Boniface, Sadie, James Kneale, and Nicola Shelton. "Drinking Pattern Is More Strongly Associated with Under-reporting of Alcohol Consumption Than Socio-Demographic Factors: Evidence from a Mixed-Methods Study." *BMC Public Health* 14 (2014): 1–9.

Boraas, Stephanie. "Volunteerism in the United States." *Monthly Labor Review* 126 (2003): 3.

Boss, P. Pauline. "Family Stress." In *Handbook of Marriage and the Family*, edited by Marvin B. Sussman and Suzanne K. Steinmetz, 725–65. New York: Springer, 1987.

Bowleg, Lisa. "When Black + Lesbian + Woman ≠ Black Lesbian Woman: The Methodological Challenges of Qualitative and Quantitative Intersectionality Research." *Sex Roles* 59 (2008): 312–25.

Brady, Jennifer, Derek K. Iwamoto, Margaux Grivel, Aylin Kaya, and Lauren Clinton. "A Systematic Review of the Salient Role of Feminine Norms on Substance Use Among Women." *Addictive Behaviors* 62 (2016): 83–90.

Brady, Kathleen T., and Susan C. Sonne. "The Role of Stress in Alcohol Use, Alcoholism Treatment, and Relapse." *Alcohol Research & Health* 23 (1999): 263–71.

Brand, Donald A., Michaela Saisana, Lisa A. Rynn, Fulvia Pennoni, and Albert B. Lowenfels. "Comparative Analysis of Alcohol Control Policies in 30 Countries." *PLoS Medicine* 4, no. 4 (2007): e15.

Brenan, Megan. "Support for Legal Marijuana Inches Up to a New High of 68%." November 9, 2020, https://news.gallup.com/poll/323582/support-legal-marijuana-inches-new-high.aspx.

Breslow, Rosalind A., I-Jen P. Castle, Chiung M. Chen, and Barry I. Graubard. "Trends in Alcohol Consumption Among Older Americans: National Health Interview Surveys, 1997 to 2014." *Alcoholism: Clinical and Experimental Research* 41 (2017): 976–86.

Briscoe, Stacy. "Direct-to-Consumer Wine Sales Up $222 Million." August 20, 2020, https://www.winemag.com/2020/08/20/wine-sales-direct-consumer.

Britton, Annie, Yoav Ben-Shlomo, Michaela Benzeval, Diana Kuh, and Steven Bell. "Life Course Trajectories of Alcohol Consumption in the United Kingdom Using Longitudinal Data from Nine Cohort Studies." *BMC Medicine* 13 (2015): 1–9.

Brofenbrenner, Urie. "Ecological Systems Theory." In *International Encyclopedia of Psychology, Vol. 3*, edited by Alan E. Kazdin, 129–33. Washington, DC: American Psychological Association, 2000.

Buckner, Julia D., Elizabeth M. Lewis, Cristina N. Abarno, Paige E. Morris, Nina I. Glover, and Michael J. Zvolensky. "Difficulties with Emotion Regulation and

Drinking During the COVID-19 Pandemic Among Undergraduates: The Serial Mediation of COVID-Related Distress and Drinking to Cope with the Pandemic." *Cognitive Behaviour Therapy* (2021): 1–15.

Buvik, Kristin. "It's Time for a Drink! Alcohol as an Investment in the Work Environment." *Drugs: Education, Prevention and Policy* 27 (2020): 86–91.

Caces, M. Fe, Thomas C. Harford, Gerald D. Williams, and Eleanor Z. Hanna. "Alcohol Consumption and Divorce Rates in the United States." *Journal of Studies on Alcohol* 60 (1999): 647–52.

Caetano, Raul, John Schafer, and Carol B. Cunradi. "Alcohol-Related Intimate Partner Violence Among White, Black, and Hispanic Couples in the United States." *Alcohol Research and Health* 25 (2001): 58–65.

Caetano, Raul, Suhasini Ramisetty-Mikler, Louise R. Floyd, and Christine McGrath. "The Epidemiology of Drinking Among Women of Child-Bearing Age." *Alcoholism: Clinical and Experimental Research* 30 (2006): 1023–30.

Calina, Daniela, Thomas Hartung, Ileana Mardare, Mihaela Mitroi, Konstantinos Poulas, Aristidis Tsatsakis, Ion Rogoveanu, and Anca Oana Docea. "COVID-19 Pandemic and Alcohol Consumption: Impacts and Interconnections." *Toxicology Reports* 8 (2021): 529–35.

Capraro, Rocco L. "Why College Men Drink: Alcohol, Adventure, and the Paradox of Masculinity." *Journal of American College Health* 48 (2000): 307–15.

Case, Anne, and Angus Deaton. "Rising Morbidity and Mortality in Midlife Among White Non-Hispanic Americans in the 21st Century." *Proceedings of the National Academy of Sciences* 112 (2015): 15078–83.

Cassetty, Samantha. "Pedialyte and Other Good Ways to Bounce Back from a Hangover." April 2, 2018, https://www.nbcnews.com/better/pop-culture/best-way -bounce-back-hangover-ncna861326.

Center for Behavioral Health Statistics and Quality. "More Than 7 Million Children Live with a Parent with Alcohol Problems." February 16, 2012, https://www.samhsa .gov/data/sites/default/files/Spot061ChildrenOfAlcoholics2012/Spot061Children OfAlcoholics2012.pdf.

Centers for Disease Control. "Alcohol and Substance Use." July 15, 2020, https://www .cdc.gov/coronavirus/2019-ncov/daily-life-coping/stress-coping/alcohol-use.html.

Chambers, Sophia E., Ellen R. Copson, Peter F. Dutey-Magni, Caspian Priest, Annie S. Anderson, and Julia M. A. Sinclair. "Alcohol Use and Breast Cancer Risk: A Qualitative Study of Women's Perspectives to Inform the Development of a Preventative Intervention in Breast Clinics." *European Journal of Cancer Care* 28 (2019): e13075.15.

Chartier, Karen G., Nathaniel S. Thomas, and Kenneth S. Kendler. "Interrelationship Between Family History of Alcoholism and Generational Status in the Prediction of Alcohol Dependence in US Hispanics." *Psychological Medicine* 47 (2017): 137–47.

Cheers, Christopher, Sarah Callinan, and Amy Pennay. "The 'Sober Eye': Examining Attitudes Towards Non-Drinkers in Australia." *Psychology and Health* 36 (2020): 385–404.

Chilcoat, Howard D., and Naomi Breslau. "Alcohol Disorders in Young Adulthood: Effects of Transitions into Adult Roles." *Journal of Health and Social Behavior* (1996): 339–49.

Cho, Young Ik, and Kathleen S. Crittenden. "The Impact of Adult Roles on Drinking Among Women in the United States." *Substance Use and Misuse* 41 (2006): 17–34.

Codazzi, Karen, Valéria Pero, and André Albuquerque Sant'Anna. "Social Norms and Female Labor Participation in Brazil." *Review of Development Economics* 22 (2018): 1513–35.

Cohen, Sheldon, and Denise Janicki-Deverts. "Who's Stressed? Distributions of Psychological Stress in the United States in Probability Samples from 1983, 2006, and 2009." *Journal of Applied Social Psychology* 42 (2012): 1320–34.

Colbert, Stephanie, Claire Wilkinson, Louise Thornton, and Robyn Richmond. "COVID-19 and Alcohol in Australia: Industry Changes and Public Health Impacts." *Drug and Alcohol Review* (2020), doi: 10.1111/dar.13092.

Connor, J. "Alcohol Consumption as a Cause of Cancer." *Addiction* 112 (2017): 222–28.

Conti, Richard P. "Family Estrangement: Establishing a Prevalence Rate." *Journal of Psychology and Behavioral Science* 3 (2015): 28–35.

Cook, Philip J. *Paying the Tab: The Costs and Benefits of Alcohol Control*. Princeton, NJ: Princeton University Press, 2007.

Cook, Won Kim, Jason Bond, and Thomas K. Greenfield. "Are Alcohol Policies Associated with Alcohol Consumption in Low- and Middle-Income Countries?" *Addiction* 109 (2014): 1081–90.

Cottrell, Sarah. "How Mommy Drinking Culture Has Normalized Alcoholism for Women in America." July 10, 2021, https://www.babble.com/parenting/mommy -drinking-culture-wine-motherhood/.

Cranwell, Jo, Magdalena Opazo-Breton, and John Britton. "Adult and Adolescent Exposure to Tobacco and Alcohol Content in Contemporary YouTube Music Videos in Great Britain: A Population Estimate." *Journal of Epidemiology and Community Health* 70 (2016): 488–92.

Curlee, Joan. "Alcoholism and the 'Empty Nest.'" *Bulletin of the Menninger Clinic* 33 (1969): 165.

Curtis, Brenda L., Samantha J. Lookatch, Danielle E. Ramo, James R. McKay, Richard S. Feinn, and Henry R. Kranzler. "Meta-Analysis of the Association of Alcohol-Related Social Media Use with Alcohol Consumption and Alcohol-Related Problems in Adolescents and Young Adults." *Alcoholism: Clinical and Experimental Research* 42 (2018): 978–86.

Czeisler, Mark É., Rashon I. Lane, Joshua F. Wiley, Charles A. Czeisler, Mark E. Howard, and Shantha M. W. Rajaratnam. "Follow-Up Survey of US Adult Reports of Mental Health, Substance Use, and Suicidal Ideation During the COVID-19 Pandemic, September 2020." *JAMA Network Open* 4 (2021): e2037665-e2037665.

Dann, Lotta. *The Wine O'Clock Myth*. Sydney, Australia: Allen & Unwin, 2021.

David, Jonathan Noel, Jane Landon, Nicole Thornton, and Tim Lobstein. "Alcohol Marketing and Youth Alcohol Consumption: A Systematic Review of Longitudinal Studies Published Since 2008." *Addiction* 112 (2017): 7–20.

Davis, Alyssa. "In U.S., Opioids Viewed as Most Serious Local Drug Problem." July 29, 2016. https://news.gallup.com/poll/194042/opioids-viewed-serious-local-drug -problem.aspx.

Davis-Berman, Jennifer. "Older Men in the Homeless Shelter: In-Depth Conversations Lead to Practice Implications." *Journal of Gerontological Social Work* 54 (2011): 456–74.

De Beauvoir, Simone. *The Second Sex*. New York: Vintage, 1989.

Dereshinsky, Julie Ward. "The Uneventful Monday Night That Made Me Stop Drinking." February 20, 2021, https://www.scarymommy.com/uneventful-monday-night -stop-drinking/.

DeWit, David J., Edward M. Adlaf, David R. Offord, and Alan C. Ogborne. "Age at First Alcohol Use: A Risk Factor for the Development of Alcohol Disorders." *American Journal of Psychiatry* 157 (2000): 745–50.

Dole, Elizabeth Hanford, Dean R. Gerstein, Steve Olson, and National Research Council. *Alcohol in America: Taking Action to Prevent Abuse*. Washington, DC: National Academies Press, 1985.

Druckerman, Sharon, and Sean Dooley. "Secret Life: Mom Confesses to Alcoholism." ABC News. April 27, 2010, https://abcnews.go.com/2020/mom-stress-mother hood-drove-drink/story?id=10488897.

Dube, Shanta R., Robert F. Anda, Vincent J. Felitti, Janet B. Croft, Valerie J. Edwards, and Wayne H. Giles. "Growing Up with Parental Alcohol Abuse: Exposure to Childhood Abuse, Neglect, and Household Dysfunction." *Child Abuse & Neglect* 25 (2001): 1627–40.

Elder, Glen H., Monica Kirkpatrick Johnson, and Robert Crosnoe. "The Emergence and Development of Life Course Theory." In *Handbook of the Life Course*, edited by J. K. Mortimer and M. J. Shanahan, 3–19. Boston, MA: Springer, 2003.

Elek, Elvira, Shelly L. Harris, Claudia M. Squire, Marjorie Margolis, Mary Kate Weber, Elizabeth Parra Dang, and Betsy Mitchell. "Women's Knowledge, Views, and Experiences Regarding Alcohol Use and Pregnancy: Opportunities to Improve Health Messages." *American Journal of Health Education* 44 (2013): 177–90.

Ephron, Nora. *I Remember Nothing*. New York: Alfred. A. Knopf, 2010.

Esser, Marissa B., Adam Sherk, Yong Liu, Timothy S. Naimi, Timothy Stockwell, Mandy Stahre, Dafna Kanny, Michael Landen, Richard Saitz, and Robert D. Brewer. "Deaths and Years of Potential Life Lost from Excessive Alcohol Use— United States, 2011–2015." *Morbidity and Mortality Weekly Report* 69 (2020): 1428.

Esser, Marissa B., Heather Clayton, Zewditu Demissie, Dafna Kanny, and Robert D. Brewer. "Current and Binge Drinking Among High School Students—United States, 1991–2015." *Morbidity and Mortality Weekly Report* 66 (2017): 474.

Esser, Marissa B., Sarra L. Hedden, Dafna Kanny, Robert D. Brewer, Joseph C. Gfroerer, and Timothy S. Naimi. "Peer Reviewed: Prevalence of Alcohol Dependence Among US Adult Drinkers, 2009–2011." *Preventing Chronic Disease* 11 (2014), doi: 10.5888%2Fpcd11.140329.

Fetters, Ashley, "The Many Faces of the 'Wine Mom.'" May 23, 2020, https://www .theatlantic.com/family/archive/2020/05/wine-moms-explained/612001.

Fingarette, Herbert. *Heavy Drinking: The Myth of Alcoholism as a Disease*. Berkeley, CA: University of California Press, 1988.

Finkelstein, Norma. "Treatment Issues for Alcohol- and Drug-Dependent Pregnant and Parenting Women." *Health & Social Work* 19 (1994): 7–15.

Fitzgerald, Niamh, Kathryn Angus, Carol Emslie, Deborah Shipton, and Linda Bauld. "Gender Differences in the Impact of Population-Level Alcohol Policy Interventions: Evidence Synthesis of Systematic Reviews." *Addiction* 111 (2016): 1735–47.

Flood, Sarah, Ann Meier, and Kelly Musick. "Reassessing Parents' Leisure Quality with Direct Measures of Well-Being: Do Children Detract from Parents' Down Time?" *Journal of Marriage and Family* 82 (2020): 1326–39.

Friedan, Betty. *The Feminine Mystique, 10th Anniversary Edition*. New York: Dell Publishing, 1974.

Freitas, Donna. *The Happiness Effect: How Social Media Is Driving a Generation to Appear Perfect at Any Cost*. Oxford, England: Oxford University Press, 2017.

Frone, Michael R. "Work Stress and Alcohol Use: Developing and Testing a Biphasic Self-Medication Model." *Work & Stress* 30 (2016): 374–94.

Frone, Michael R., Grace M. Barnes, and Michael P. Farrell. "Relationship of Work-Family Conflict to Substance Use Among Employed Mothers: The Role of Negative Affect." *Journal of Marriage and the Family* (1994): 1019–30.

Frone, Michael R., Marcia Russell, and M. Lynne Cooper. "Relationship of Work-Family Conflict, Gender, and Alcohol Expectancies to Alcohol Use/Abuse." *Journal of Organizational Behavior* 14 (1993): 545–58.

Gallup. "Alcohol and Drinking." May 20, 2021, https://news.gallup.com/poll/1582/alcohol-drinking.aspx.

GBD 2016 Alcohol Collaborators. "Alcohol Use and Burden for 195 Countries and Territories, 1990–2016: A Systematic Analysis for the Global Burden of Disease Study 2016." *The Lancet* 392 (2018): 1015–35.

Ge, Lixia, Chun Wei Yap, Reuben Ong, and Bee Hoon Heng. "Social Isolation, Loneliness and Their Relationships with Depressive Symptoms: A Population-Based Study," *PLoS One* 12 (2017): e0182145.

Geiger, A. W., Gretchen Livingston, and Kristen Bialik. "6 Facts About U.S. Moms." Accessed May 8, 2019, https://www.pewresearch.org/fact-tank/2019/05/08/facts-about-u-s-mothers.

Giangreco, Leigh. "At D.C.'s Liquor Stores, Sales Have Doubled and a Whole Lot of Everclear Is Flying Off the Shelves." March 16, 2020, https://dcist.com/story/20/03/16/at-d-c-s-liquor-stores-sales-have-doubled-and-a-whole-lot-of-everclear-is-flying-off-the-shelves/.

Gillespie, Claire. "Mommy Doesn't Need Wine: The Stigma of Being a Sober Mother." July 24, 2018, https://www.thefix.com/mommy-doesnt-need-wine-stigma-being-sober-mother.

Glaser, Gabrielle. *Her Best Kept Secret*. New York: Simon & Schuster, 2013.

Glynn, Sarah Jane. "Breadwinning Mothers Continue to Be the U.S. Norm." May 10, 2019, https://www.americanprogress.org/issues/women/reports/2019/05/10/469739/breadwinning-mothers-continue-u-s-norm/.

Goffman, Erving. *The Presentation of Self in Everyday Life*. Garden City, NY: Doubleday Anchor Books, 1959.

Gomberg, Edith L., "Risk Factors for Drinking over a Woman's Life Span." *Alcohol Health and Research World* 18 (1994): 220.

Gomberg, Edith L. "Women and Alcohol: Use and Abuse." *Journal of Nervous and Mental Disease* 181 (1993): 211–19.

Gomberg, Edith L. "Women and Alcoholism: Psychosocial Issues." *Research Monograph* 16 (1986): 78–120.

Grall, Timothy. "Custodial Mothers and Fathers and Their Child Support: 2017." May 2020, https://www.census.gov/content/dam/Census/library/publications/2020/demo/p60-269.pdf.

Grant, Bridget F., S. Patricia Chou, Tulshi D. Saha, Roger P. Pickering, Bradley T. Kerridge, W. June Ruan, Boji Huang, Jeesun Jung, Haitao Zhang, Amy Fan, and Deborah S. Hasin. "Prevalence of 12-Month Alcohol Use, High-Risk Drinking, And DSM-IV Alcohol Use Disorder in The United States, 2001–2002 to 2012–2013: Results from the National Epidemiologic Survey on Alcohol and Related Conditions." *JAMA Psychiatry* 74 (2017): 911–23.

Grant, Bridget F., Risë B. Goldstein, Tulshi D. Saha, S. Patricia Chou, Jeesun Jung, Haitao Zhang, Roger P. Pickering, June Ruan, Sharon M. Smith, Boji Huang, and Deborah S. Hasin. "Epidemiology of DSM-5 Alcohol Use Disorder: Results from the National Epidemiologic Survey on Alcohol and Related Conditions III." *JAMA Psychiatry* 72 (2015): 757–66.

Grant, Bridget F., Frederick S. Stinson, and Thomas C. Harford. "Age at Onset of Alcohol Use and DSM-IV Alcohol Abuse and Dependence: A 12-Year Follow-Up." *Journal of Substance Abuse* 13 (2001): 493–504.

Griffin, Christine. "Good Girls, Bad Girls: Anglocentrism and Diversity in the Constitution of Contemporary Girlhood." In *All About the Girl: Culture, Power, and Identity*, edited by Anita Harris, 29–43. New York: Routledge, 2004.

Grucza, Richard A., Kenneth J. Sher, William C. Kerr, Melissa J. Krauss, Camillia K. Lui, Yoanna E. McDowell, Sarah Hartz, Gurpal Virdi, and Laura J. Bierut. "Trends in Adult Alcohol Use and Binge Drinking in the Early 21st-Century United States: A Meta-Analysis of 6 National Survey Series." *Alcoholism: Clinical and Experimental Research* 42 (2018): 1939–50.

Grzywacz, Joseph G., and Nadine F. Marks. "Family, Work, Work-Family Spillover, and Problem Drinking During Midlife." *Journal of Marriage and Family* 62 (2000): 336–48.

Harper's Bazaar. "Anne Hathaway on Giving Up Alcohol: 'It's Irritating How Well It's Going," April 24, 2019, https://www.harpersbazaar.com/uk/celebrities/news/a27249916/anne-hathaway-giving-up-alcohol/.

Harris, Anita. "Jamming Girl Culture: Young Women and Consumer Citizenship." In *All About the Girl: Culture, Power, and Identity*, edited by Anita Harris, 163–72. New York: Routledge, 2004.

Haydon, Helen M., Patricia L. Obst, and Ioni Lewis. "Beliefs Underlying Women's Intentions to Consume Alcohol." *BMC Women's Health* 16 (2016): 1–12.

Hayes, Sharon. *The Cultural Contradictions of Motherhood*. New Haven, CT: Yale University Press, 1998.

Heil, Emily. "The Key to White Claw's Surging Popularity: Marketing to a Post-Gender World." September 9, 2019, https://www.washingtonpost.com/news /voraciously/wp/2019/09/10/the-key-to-white-claws-surging-popularity-market ing-to-a-post-gender-world/.

Henderson, Cydney. "Chrissy Teigen Explains Why She Quit Drinking, Praises Book That Inspired Lifestyle Change." December 31, 2020, https://www.usatoday.com /story/entertainment/celebrities/2020/12/31/chrissy-teigen-reveals-shes-4-weeks -sober-why-she-quit-drinking/4097801001.

Hendriks, Hanneke, Danii Wilmsen, Wim Van Dalen, and Winifred A. Gebhardt. "Picture Me Drinking: Alcohol-Related Posts by Instagram Influencers Popular Among Adolescents and Young Adults." *Frontiers in Psychology* 10 (2020): 2991.

Hill, Reuben. *Families Under Stress*. New York: Harper & Row, 1949.

History.com. "War on Drugs." December 17, 2019, https://www.history.com/topics /crime/the-war-on-drugs#section_5.

Hochschild, Arlie, *The Second Shift*. New York: Avon Books, 1989.

Hollenstein, Jenna. *Drinking to Distraction*. Morrisville, NC: Lulu Publishing, 2014.

Hook, Jennifer L. "Women's Housework: New Tests of Time and Money." *Journal of Marriage and Family* 79 (2017): 179–98.

Howorth, Claire. "Motherhood Is Hard to Get Wrong. So Why Do so Many Moms Feel so Bad About Themselves?" October 19, 2017, http://time.com/magazine /us/4989032/october-30th-2017-vol-190-no-18-u-s.

Hrynowski, Zach. "What Percentage of Americans Smoke Marijuana?" July 2019, https://news.gallup.com/poll/284135/percentage-americans-smoke-marijuana .aspx.

Ianzito, Christina C. "Alcohol Use on the Rise During Pandemic." April 17, 2020, https://aarp.org/health/healthy-living/info-2020/coronavirus-alcohol.html.

Infurna, Frank J., Denis Gerstorf, and Margie E. Lachman. "Midlife in the 2020s: Opportunities and Challenges." *American Psychologist* 75 (2020): 470.

Institute of Alcohol Studies. "Changing Trends in Women's Drinking." September 22, 2017, http://www.ias.org.uk/Alcohol-knowledge-centre/Alcohol-and-women /Factsheets/The-effects-of-alcohol-on-women.aspx.

Institute of Alcohol Studies. "The Effects of Alcohol on Women." September 22, 2017, http://www.ias.org.uk/Alcohol-knowledge-centre/Alcohol-and-women/Fact sheets/Changing-trends-in-womens-drinking.aspx.

Institute of Alcohol Studies. "Why Are Women Drinking More?" September 22, 2017, http://www.ias.org.uk/Alcohol-knowledge-centre/Alcohol-and-women/Factsheets /Why-are-women-drinking-more.aspx.

Ishii-Kuntz, Masako. "Social Interaction and Psychological Well-Being: Comparison Across Stages of Adulthood." *The International Journal of Aging and Human Development* 30 (1990): 15–36.

Jersild, Devon. *Happy Hours: Alcohol in a Woman's Life*. New York: Harper, 2021.

Johnson, Fred W., Paul J. Gruenewald, Andrew J. Treno, and Gail Armstong Taff. "Drinking Over the Life Course within Gender and Ethnic Groups: A Hyperparametric Analysis." *Journal of Studies on Alcohol* 59 (1998): 568–80.

Johnston, Lloyd D., Richard A. Miech, Patrick M. O'Malley, Jerald G. Bachman, John E. Schulenberg, and Megan E. Patrick. *Monitoring the Future National Survey Results on Drug Use, 1975–2017: Overview, Key Findings on Adolescent Drug Use.* Ann Arbor, MI: Institute for Social Research, University of Michigan, 2018.

Jones, Jeffrey M. "Drinking Highest Among Educated Upper-Income Americans." July 27, 2015, http://www.gallup.com/poll/184358/drinking-highest-among-edu cated-upper-income-americans.aspx.

Jones, Jeffrey M. "Most in U.S. Say Consuming Alcohol, Marijuana Morally OK." June 4, 2018, https://news.gallup.com/poll/235250/say-consuming-alcohol-mari juana-morally.aspx.

Jones, Jeffrey M. "U.S. Drinkers Divide Between Beer and Wine as Favorite." August 1, 2013, http://www.gallup.com/poll/163787/drinkers-divide-beer-wine-favorite .aspx.

Jones, Sandra C., and Chloe S. Gordon. "A Systematic Review of Children's Alcohol-Related Knowledge, Attitudes and Expectancies." *Preventive Medicine* 105 (2017): 19–31.

Kamp Dush, Claire M., Jill E. Yavorsky, and Sarah J. Schoppe-Sullivan. "What Are Men Doing While Women Perform Extra Unpaid Labor? Leisure and Specialization at the Transitions to Parenthood." *Sex Roles* 78 (2018): 715–30.

Keating, Dan. "Nine Charts That Show How White Women are Drinking Themselves to Death." December 23, 2016, https://www.washingtonpost.com/news /national/wp/2016/12/23/nine-charts-that-show-how-white-women-are-drinking -themselves-to-death/?utm_term=.0b32805e061e.

Keating, Dan, and Kennedy Elliott. "Why Death Rates for White Women in Rural America Are Spiking." April 9, 2016, https://www.washingtonpost.com/graphics /national/white-death/.

Keating, Dan, Kennedy Elliott, and Leslie Shapiro. "White Women Are Dying Faster All Over America—But What About Where You Live?" September 22, 2017, https://www.washingtonpost.com/graphics/national/death-rates-your-county/.

Kehily, Mary Jane. "Taking Centre Stage? Girlhood and the Contradictions of Femininity Across Three Generations." *Girlhood Studies* 1 (2008): 51–71.

Kelly, John F., and Bettina B. Hoeppner. "Does Alcoholics Anonymous Work Differently for Men and Women? A Moderated Multiple-Mediation Analysis in a Large Clinical Sample." *Drug and Alcohol Dependence* 130 (2013): 186–93.

Kendler, K. S., H. Ohlsson, J. Sundquist, and K. Sundquist. "Transmission of Alcohol Use Disorder Across Three Generations: A Swedish National Study." *Psychological Medicine* 48 (2018): 33.

Kerr, William C., Camillia K. Lui, Edwina Williams, Yu Ye, Thomas K. Greenfield, and E. Anne Lown. "Health Risk Factors Associated with Lifetime Abstinence from Alcohol in the 1979 National Longitudinal Survey of Youth Cohort." *Alcoholism: Clinical and Experimental Research* 41 (2017): 388–98.

Kerr, William C., Thomas K. Greenfield, Jason Bond, Yu Ye, and Jürgen Rehm. "Age-Period-Cohort Modelling of Alcohol Volume and Heavy Drinking Days in the US National Alcohol Surveys: Divergence in Younger and Older Adult Trends." *Addiction* 104 (2009): 27–37.

Kerr-Corrêa, Florence, Andrea M. Hegedus, Luzia A. Trinca, Adriana M. Tucci, Ligia R. S. Kerr-Pontes, and A. F. Sanches. "Differences in Drinking Patterns Between Men and Women in Brazil." In *Alcohol, Gender and Drinking Problems*, edited by Isidore S. Obat and Robin Room, 49–68. Geneva, Switzerland: World Health Organization, 2005.

Keyes, Katherine M., and Richard Miech. "Age, Period, and Cohort Effects in Heavy Episodic Drinking in the US from 1985 to 2009." *Drug and Alcohol Dependence* 132 (2013): 140–48.

Killingsworth, Ben. "'Drinking Stories' from a Playgroup: Alcohol in the Lives of Middle-Class Mothers in Australia." *Ethnography* 7 (2006): 357–84, 372, 375.

Kindy, Kennedy, and Dan Keating. "For Women, Heavy Drinking Has Been Normalized. That's Dangerous." December 23, 2016, https://www.washingtonpost.com/national/for-women-heavy-drinking-has-been-normalized-thats-dangerous/2016/12/23/0e701120-c381-11e6-9578-0054287507db_story.html?utm_term=.6840ab0d9bc2.

Kleinand, Laura F., and Lillian A. Ackerman. *Women and Power in Native North America*. Norman, OK: University of Oklahoma Press, 1995.

Knepper, Cheryl. "Women and the Impact of Addiction: Special Issues in Treatment and Recovery." July 2012, https://www.naatp.org/sites/naatp.org/files/wp-content/uploads/2012/07/Knepper-Women-Presentation.pdf .

Kreager, Derek A., Ross L. Matsueda, and Elena A. Erosheva. "Motherhood and Criminal Desistance in Disadvantaged Neighborhoods." *Criminology* 48 (2010): 221–58.

Kuntsche, Emmanuel. "'Do Grown-Ups Become Happy When They Drink?' Alcohol Expectancies Among Preschoolers." *Experimental and Clinical Psychopharmacology* 25 (2017): 24.

Laborde, Nicole D., and Christina Mair. "Alcohol Use Patterns Among Postpartum Women." *Maternal and Child Health Journal* 16 (2012): 1810–19.

Landrine, Hope, Stephen Bardwell, and Tina Dean. "Gender Expectations for Alcohol Use: A Study of the Significance of the Masculine Role." *Sex Roles* 19 (1988): 703–12.

Lechner, William V., Natasha K. Sidhu, Jackson T. Jin, Ahmad A. Kittaneh, Kimberly R. Laurene, and Deric R. Kenne. "Increases in Risky Drinking During the COVID-19 Pandemic Assessed via Longitudinal Cohort Design: Associations with Racial Tensions, Financial Distress, Psychological Distress and Virus-Related Fears." *Alcohol and Alcoholism* (2021), doi: 10.1093/alcalc/agab019.

Leonard, Kenneth E., and Rina D. Eiden. "Marital and Family Processes in the Context of Alcohol Use and Alcohol Disorders." *Annual Review of Clinical Psychology* 3 (2007): 285–310.

Liang, Linda A., Ursula Berger, and Christian Brand. "Psychosocial Factors Associated with Symptoms of Depression, Anxiety and Stress Among Single Mothers with Young Children: A Population-Based Study." *Journal of Affective Disorders* 242 (2019): 255–64.

Linden, Audrey, and Sillence, Elizabeth. "'I'm Finally Allowed to Be Me': Parent-Child Estrangement and Psychological Wellbeing." *Families, Relationships and Societies* 10 (2021): 325–41, doi: 10.1332/204674319x15647593365505.

Lipari, Rachel N., and Struther L. Van Horn. "Children Living with Parents Who Have a Substance Use Disorder." *The CBHSQ Report*. August 24, 2017, https://www.ncbi.nlm.nih.gov/books/NBK464590/.

Littler, Jo. "Mothers Behaving Badly: Chaotic Hedonism and the Crisis of Neoliberal Social Reproduction." *Cultural Studies* 34 (2020): 499–520.

Livingston, Gretchen. "More Than One-in-Ten U.S. Parents Are Also Caring for an Adult." November 29, 2018, https://www.pewresearch.org/fact-tank/2018/11/29/more-than-one-in-ten-u-s-parents-are-also-caring-for-an-adult.

Livingston, Michael, and Sarah Callinan. "Underreporting in Alcohol Surveys: Whose Drinking Is Underestimated?" *Journal of Studies on Alcohol and Drugs* 76 (2015): 158–64.

Lye, Diane N. "Adult Child–Parent Relationships." *Annual Review of Sociology* 22 (1996): 79–102.

Lyons, Antonia C., and Sara A. Willott. "Alcohol Consumption, Gender Identities and Women's Changing Social Positions." *Sex Roles* 59 (2008): 694–712.

Mark, Tami L., Cheryl A. Kassed, Rita Vandivort-Warren, Katharine R. Levit, and Henry R. Kranzler. "Alcohol and Opioid Dependence Medications: Prescription Trends, Overall and by Physician Specialty." *Drug and Alcohol Dependence* 99 (2009): 345–49.

Marshal, Michael P. "For Better or for Worse? The Effects of Alcohol Use on Marital Functioning." *Clinical Psychology Review* 23 (2003): 959–97.

Martin, Jack K., Joan M. Kraft, and Paul M. Roman. "Extent and Impact of Alcohol and Drug Use Problems in the Workplace." In *Drug Testing in the Workplace,* edited by Scott Macdonald and Paul Roman, 3–31. Boston, MA: Springer, 1994.

Maume, David J., Rachel A. Sebastian, and Anthony R. Bardo. "Gender, Work-Family Responsibilities, and Sleep." *Gender & Society* 24 (2010): 746–68.

Mayrhofer, Mira, and Jörg Matthes. "Drinking at Work: The Portrayal of Alcohol in Workplace-Related TV Dramas." *Mass Communication and Society* 21 (2018): 94–114.

McCarthy, Jane Ribbens, Val Gillies, and Carol-Ann Hooper. "'Family Troubles' and 'Troubling Families': Opening Up Fertile Ground." *Journal of Family Issues* 40 (2019): 2207–224.

McCrady, Barbara S., Elizabeth E. Epstein, and Kathryn F. Fokas. "Treatment Interventions for Women with Alcohol Use Disorder." *Alcohol Research: Current Reviews* 40 (2020), doi: 10.35946%2Farcr.v40.2.08.

McCubbin, Hamilton I., Constance B. Joy, A. Elizabeth Cauble, Joan K. Comeau, Joan M. Patterson, and Richard H. Needle. "Family Stress and Coping: A Decade Review." *Journal of Marriage and the Family* 42 (1980): 855–71.

McFarlin, Susan K., and William Fals-Stewart. "Workplace Absenteeism and Alcohol Use: A Sequential Analysis." *Psychology of Addictive Behaviors* 16 (2002): 17.

McKetta, Sarah, and Katherine M. Keyes. "Heavy and Binge Alcohol Drinking and Parenting Status in the United States from 2006 to 2018: An Analysis of Nationally Representative Cross-Sectional Surveys." *PLoS Medicine* 16 (2019): e1002954.

Measham, Fiona. "'Doing Gender'—'Doing Drugs': Conceptualizing the Gendering of Drugs Cultures." *Contemporary Drug Problems* 29 (2002): 335–73.

Mellinger, Jessica L., Kerby Shedden, Gerald Scott Winder, Elliot Tapper, Megan Adams, Robert J. Fontana, Michael L. Volk, Frederic C. Blow, and Anna S. F. Lok. "The High Burden of Alcoholic Cirrhosis in Privately Insured Persons in the United States." *Hepatology* 68 (2018): 872–82.

Milic, Jelena, Marija Glisic, Trudy Voortman, Laura Pletsch Borba, Eralda Asllanaj, Lyda Z. Rojas, Jenna Troup, et al. "Menopause, Aging, and Alcohol Use Disorders in Women." *Maturitas* 111 (2018): 100–9.

Miller, Korin. "Pedialyte's New Powder Packets Are Basically Made for Adult Hangovers." December 27, 2018, https://www.womenshealthmag.com/health/a25694156/pedialyte-packets-for-hangovers.

Miller-Tutzauer, Carol, Kenneth E. Leonard, and Michael Windle. "Marriage and Alcohol Use: A Longitudinal Study of 'Maturing Out.'" *Journal of Studies on Alcohol* 52 (1991): 434–40.

Milne, Ben. "How Babycham Changed British Drinking Habits." December 23, 2013, https://www.bbc.com/news/magazine-25302633.

Mintel Press Office. "Alcohol Manufacturers Drink in Profits from At-Home Consumption, Reports Mintel." July 15, 2010, https://www.mintel.com/press-centre/food-and-drink/alcohol-manufacturers-drink-in-profits-from-at-home-consumption-reports-mintel#:~:text=Among%20alcohol%20drinkers%2C%2090%25%20consume,5.7.

Moreno, Megan A., and Jennifer M. Whitehill. "Influence of Social Media on Alcohol Use in Adolescents and Young Adults." *Alcohol Research: Current Reviews* 36 (2014): 91.

Moreno, Megan A., Laina Mercer, Henry N. Young, Elizabeth D. Cox, and Bradley Kerr. "Testing Young Adults' Reactions to Facebook Cues and Their Associations with Alcohol Use." *Substance Use and Misuse* 54 (2019): 1450–60.

Mudar, Pamela, Jill N. Kearns, and Kenneth E. Leonard. "The Transition to Marriage and Changes in Alcohol Involvement Among Black Couples and White Couples." *Journal of Studies on Alcohol* 63 (2002): 568–76.

Muthén, Bengt O., and Linda K. Muthén. "The Development of Heavy Drinking and Alcohol-Related Problems from Ages 18 to 37 in a US National Sample." *Journal of Studies on Alcohol* 61 (2000): 290–300.

Nam, Su-Jung. "Mediating Effect of Social Support on the Relationship Between Older Adults' Use of Social Media and Their Quality-of-Life." *Current Psychology* (2019): 1–9.

National Institute of Alcohol Abuse and Alcoholism (NIAAA). "Alcohol Facts and Statistics." June 4, 2021, https://www.niaaa.nih.gov/publications/brochures-and-fact-sheets/alcohol-facts-and-statistics.

NIAAA. "Alcohol Use Disorder: A Comparison Between DSM-IV and DSM-5." July 7, 2020, https://www.niaaa.nih.gov/publications/brochures-and-fact-sheets /alcohol-use-disorder-comparison-between-dsm.

NIAAA. "Recommended Alcohol Questions." July 10, 2020, https://www.niaaa.nih .gov/research/guidelines-and-resources/recommended-alcohol-questions.

NIAAA. *10th Special Report to the US Congress on Alcohol and Health from the Secretary of Health and Human Services.* June 2000, https://pubs.niaaa.nih.gov/pu blications/10report/10thspecialreport.pdf.

National Institute on Drug Abuse. "Monitoring the Future." December 18, 2019, https://www.drugabuse.gov/drug-topics/trends-statistics/infographics/monitoring -future-2019-survey-results-overall-findings.

Neger, Emily N., and Ronald J. Prinz. "Interventions to Address Parenting and Parental Substance Abuse: Conceptual and Methodological Considerations." *Clinical Psychology Review* 39 (2015): 71–82.

Nesi, Jacqueline W., Andrew Rothenberg, Andrea M. Hussong, and Kristina M. Jackson. "Friends' Alcohol-Related Social Networking Site Activity Predicts Escalations in Adolescent Drinking: Mediation by Peer Norms." *Journal of Adolescent Health* 60 (2017): 641–47.

Newman, Katelyn. "A Different Dose of Drug Education." November 14, 2019, https://www.usnews.com/news/healthiest-communities/articles/2019-11-14/high -school-drug-curriculum-includes-harm-reduction-emphasis.

Nicholls, Emily. *Negotiating Femininities in the Neoliberal Night-Time Economy: Too Much of a Girl?* Cham, Switzerland: Springer, 2018.

Nicogossian, Claire. "Hoda & Jenna, Please Get Rid of the Wine." July 31, 2019, https://community.today.com/parentingteam/post/hoda-jenna-please-get-rid-of -the-wine.

Nielsen, Samara Joy. "Calories Consumed from Alcoholic Beverages by US Adults, 2007–2010." November 2012, https://www.cdc.gov/nchs/products/databriefs /db110.htm.

Nielsen. "Rebalancing the 'COVID-19 Effect' on Alcohol Sales." May 7, 2020, https://www.nielsen.com/us/en/insights/article/2020/rebalancing-the-covid-19 -effect-on-alcohol-sales.

Nolen-Hoeksema, Susan, and Lori M. Hilt. "Gender Differences in Depression." *Current Directions in Psychological Science* 10 (2009): 173–76.

Norman, Philip. *Babycham Night.* London: Pan Publishing, 2011.

OECD. *Tackling Harmful Alcohol Use.* May 12, 2015, https://www.oecd.org/health /tackling-harmful-alcohol-use-9789264181069-en.htm.

Park, Robert Ezra, and Ernest Watson Burgess. *Introduction to the Science of Sociology.* Glasgow, Scotland: Good Press, 2019.

Parramore, Lynn Stuart. "'Promising Young Woman': Covid and the Women Giving Up Alcohol to Fight the Patriarchy." January 31, 2021, https://www.nbcnews .com/think/opinion/promising-young-woman-covid-women-giving-alcohol-fight -patriarchy-ncna1256229.

Passias, Emily J., Liana Sayer, and Joanna R. Pepin. "Who Experiences Leisure Deficits? Mothers' Marital Status and Leisure Time." *Journal of Marriage and Family* 79 (2017): 1001–22.

Pearson, Matthew R., Megan Kirouac, and Katie Witkiewitz. "Questioning the Validity of the 4+/5+ Binge or Heavy Drinking Criterion in College and Clinical Populations." *Addiction* 111 (2016): 1720–26.

Pelletiere, Nicole. "'A Pump-and-Dump Kind of Day': How Wine-Mom Culture Shifted from Funny Memes to Unhappy Hangovers." September 6, 2019, https://www.goodmorningamerica.com/family/story/pump-dump-kind-day-wine-mom-culture-shifted-62625309.

Pepin, Joanna R., Liana C. Sayer, and Lynne M. Casper. "Marital Status and Mothers' Time Use: Childcare, Housework, Leisure, and Sleep." *Demography* 55 (2018): 107–33.

Petri, Anette Lykke, Anne Tjønneland, Michael Gamborg, Ditte Johansen, Susanne Høidrup, Thorkild I. A. Sørensen, and Morten Grønbæk. "Alcohol Intake, Type of Beverage, and Risk of Breast Cancer in Pre- and Postmenopausal Women." *Alcoholism: Clinical and Experimental Research* 28 (2004): 1084–90.

Petrzelka, Peggy, and Susan E. Mannon. "Keepin' This Little Town Going: Gender and Volunteerism in Rural America." *Gender & Society* 20 (2006): 236–58.

Pollard, Michael S., Joan S. Tucker, and Harold D. Green. "Changes in Adult Alcohol Use and Consequences During the COVID-19 Pandemic in the US." *JAMA Network Open* 3 (2020): e2022942-e2022942.

Poorman, Elisabeth. "How We Doctors Are Failing Our Patients Who Drink Too Much." March 21, 2017, http://www.wbur.org/commonhealth/2017/03/31/not-alcholic-drink-heavily.

Putney, Norella M., and Vern L. Bengtson. "Intergenerational Relations in Changing Times." In *Handbook of the Life Course*, edited by J. K. Mortimer and M. J. Shanahan, 149–64. Boston, MA: Springer, 2003.

Quora. "What Is the Intersection Theory in Sociology?" Accessed June 12, 2021, https://www.quora.com/What-is-the-intersection-theory-in-sociology.

Raine, Pamela. *Women's Perspectives on Drugs and Alcohol: The Vicious Circle*. Farnham, UK: Ashgate Publishing, 2001.

Reczek, Corinne, Tetyana Pudrovska, Deborah Carr, Mieke Beth Thomeer, and Debra Umberson. "Marital Histories and Heavy Alcohol Use Among Older Adults." *Journal of Health and Social Behavior* 57 (2016): 77–96.

Ricciardelli, Lina A., Jason P. Connor, Robert J. Williams, and Ross M. Young. "Gender Stereotypes and Drinking Cognitions as Indicators of Moderate and High Risk Drinking Among Young Women and Men." *Drug and Alcohol Dependence* 61 (2001): 129–36.

Ridley, Nicole J., Brian Draper, and Adrienne Withall. "Alcohol-Related Dementia: An Update of the Evidence." *Alzheimer's Research & Therapy* 5 (2013): 1–8.

Riemer, Abigail R., Sarah J. Gervais, Jeanine L. M. Skorinko, Sonya Maria Douglas, Heather Spencer, Katherine Nugai, Anastasia Karapanagou, and Andreas Miles-Novelo. "She Looks Like She'd Be an Animal in Bed: Dehumanization of Drinking Women in Social Contexts." *Sex Roles* 80 (2019): 617–29.

Roberts, Mary Lee A., and Martin Schiavenato, "Othering in the Nursing Context: A Concept Analysis." *Nursing Open* 4 (2017): 174–81.

Romo, Lynsey K., Dana R. Dinsmore, Tara L. Connolly, and Christine N. Davis. "An Examination of How Professionals Who Abstain from Alcohol Communicatively Negotiate Their Non-Drinking Identity." *Journal of Applied Communication Research* 43 (2015): 91–111.

Sartor, Carolyn E., Michael T. Lynskey, Kathleen K. Bucholz, Pamela A. F. Madden, Nicholas G. Martin, and Andrew C. Heath. "Timing of First Alcohol Use and Alcohol Dependence: Evidence of Common Genetic Influences." *Addiction* 104 (2009): 1512–18.

Sayer, Liana C. "Parenthood and Leisure Time Disparities." In *Contemporary Parenting and Parenthood: From News Headlines to New Research*, edited by Michelle Y. Janning, 168–98. Santa Barbara, CA: ABC-CLIO, 2018.

Scagell, Julie. "Someone Invented Wine Juice Boxes Because We Deserve to Be Happy." May 15, 2019, https://www.scarymommy.com/high-key-portable-wine -pouches.

Scary Mommy. "Scary Mommy Confessions: When You're a Mom Who Drinks." August 13, 2016, https://www.scarymommy.com/mothering-drinking.

Scharp, Kristina M., and Elizabeth Dorrance Hall. "Family Marginalization, Alienation, and Estrangement: Questioning the Nonvoluntary Status of Family Relationships." *Annals of the International Communication Association* 41 (2017): 28–45.

Scheller, Alissa. "Here Are the Rules to Buying Alcohol in Each State's Grocery Stores." August 26, 2014, updated December 6, 2017, https://www.huffingtonpost .com/2014/08/26/here-are-all-the-states-t_n_5710135.html.

Schrempft, Stephanie, Marta Jackowska, Mark Hamer, and Andrew Steptoe. "Associations Between Social Isolation, Loneliness, and Objective Physical Activity in Older Men and Women." *BMC Public Health* 19 (2019): 1–10.

Settembre, Jeanette. "Pedialyte Is the Hottest Hangover Cure, but Does It Really Work?" December 31, 2018, https://www.marketwatch.com/story/pedialyte-is-the -hottest-hangover-cure-but-does-it-really-work-2018-12-31.

Shaffer, Anne, and Byron Egeland. "Intergenerational Transmission of Familial Boundary Dissolution: Observations and Psychosocial Outcomes in Adolescence." *Family Relations* 60 (2011): 290–302.

Sharmin, Sonia, Kypros Kypri, Masuma Khanam, Monika Wadolowski, Raimondo Bruno, John Attia, Elizabeth Holliday, Kerrin Palazzi, and Richard P. Mattick. "Effects of Parental Alcohol Rules on Risky Drinking and Related Problems in Adolescence: Systematic Review and Meta-Analysis." *Drug and Alcohol Dependence* 178 (2017): 243–56.

Slade, Tim, Cath Chapman, Wendy Swift, Katherine Keyes, Zoe Tonks, and Maree Teesson. "Birth Cohort Trends in the Global Epidemiology of Alcohol Use and Alcohol-Related Harms in Men and Women: Systematic Review and Metaregression." *BMJ Open* 6 (2016), doi: 10.1136/bmjopen-2016-011827.

Smit, Koen, Carmen Voogt, Roy Otten, Marloes Kleinjan, and Emmanuel Kuntsche. "Exposure to Parental Alcohol Use Rather Than Parental Drinking Shapes Offspring's Alcohol Expectancies." *Alcoholism: Clinical and Experimental Research* 43 (2019): 1967–77.

Smith, Lorraine. "Invited Review: Help Seeking in Alcohol-Dependent Females." *Alcohol and Alcoholism* 27 (1992): 3–9.

Steiner, Allison M., and Paula C. Fletcher. "Sandwich Generation Caregiving: A Complex and Dynamic Role." *Journal of Adult Development* 24 (2017): 133–43.

Stewart, Susan D. "COVID-19, Coronavirus-Related Anxiety, and Changes in Women's Alcohol Use." *Gynecology and Women's Health* (2021), doi: 10.19080 /JGWH.2021.21.556057.

Stewart, Susan D., Gloria Jones-Johnson, and Cassandra Dorius. "Mothers' Alcohol Use When the Children Leave the Nest: An Intersectional Approach." Presentation, Midwest Sociological Society, Chicago, IL, April 17–20, 2019.

Stewart, Susan D., Gloria Jones-Johnson, and Cassandra Dorius. "Women and Alcohol Use Over the Lifecourse." Presentation, American Sociological Association, New York, August 10–13, 2019.

Stone, Andrea L., Linda G. Becker, Alice M. Huber, and Richard F. Catalano. "Review of Risk and Protective Factors of Substance Use and Problem Use in Emerging Adulthood." *Addictive Behaviors* 37 (2012): 747–75.

Sudhinaraset, May, Christina Wigglesworth, and David T. Takeuchi. "Social and Cultural Contexts of Alcohol Use: Influences in a Social-Ecological Framework." *Alcohol Research: Current Reviews* 38 (2016): 35–45.

Swartz, Kyle. "9 Trends Driving Wine Sales in 2016." January 26, 2016, http://bever agedynamics.com/2016/01/26/9-trends-driving-wine-sales-in-2016.

Tapper, Elliot B., and Neehar D. Parikh. "Mortality Due to Cirrhosis and Liver Cancer in the United States, 1999–2016: Observational Study." *BMJ* 362 (2018), doi: 10.1136/bmj.k2817.

Taylor, Zoe E., and Rand D. Conger. "Promoting Strengths and Resilience in Single-mother Families." *Child Development* 88 (2017): 350–58.

Thistle, Susan. *From Marriage to the Market: The Transformation of Women's Lives and Work*. Berkeley, CA: University of California Press, 2006.

Thoits, Peggy A. "Mechanisms Linking Social Ties and Support to Physical and Mental Health." *Journal of Health and Social Behavior* 52 (2011): 145–61.

Tiffany, Kaitlyn. "How Pedialyte Got Pedialit." September 10, 2018, https://www.vox .com/the-goods/2018/9/10/17819358/pedialyte-hangover-marketing-strategy -instagram-influencers.

Thrul, Johannes, and Emmanuel Kuntsche. "Interactions Between Drinking Motives and Friends in Predicting Young Adults' Alcohol Use." *Prevention Science* 17 (2016): 626–35.

Trickey, Erick. "Inside the Story of America's 19th-Century Opiate Addiction." January 4, 2018, https://www.smithsonianmag.com/history/inside-story-americas-19th -century-opiate-addiction-180967673.

Triggs, Charlotte. "Jenna Bush Hager Says Laura Bush Is Not a Fan of Her Today Show Day-Drinking: 'My Mom Judges.'" February 26, 2019, https://people.com /tv/jenna-bush-hager-mom-laura-bush-not-fan-today-show-wine.

Tsai, Jack, Eric B. Elbogen, Minda Huang, Carol S. North, and Robert H. Pietrzak. "Psychological Distress and Alcohol Use Disorder During the COVID-19 Era Among Middle- and Low-Income US Adults." *Journal of Affective Disorders* 288 (2021): 41–9.

Turner, Sarah, and Lucy Rocca. *The Sober Revolution: Women Calling Time on Wine O'Clock*. Abercynon, Wales: Accent Press Ltd., 2013.

U.S. Bureau of Labor Statistics. "Highlights of Women's Earnings in 2019." December 2020, https://www.bls.gov/opub/reports/womens-earnings/2019/pdf/home.pdf.

U.S. Bureau of Labor Statistics. "Labor Force Statistics from the Current Population Survey." February 12, 2021, https://www.bls.gov/opub/reports/womens-earnings/2019/pdf/home.pdf.

U.S. Census Bureau. "America's Families and Living Arrangements: 2019." 2019, https://www.census.gov/data/tables/2019/demo/families/cps-2019.html.

U.S. Census Bureau. "U.S. Census Bureau Releases 2018 Families and Living Arrangements Tables." November 14, 2018, https://www.census.gov/newsroom/press-releases/2018/families.html.

U.S. Department of Health and Human Services. "Alcohol: A Women's Health Issue." July 10, 2020, https://pubs.niaaa.nih.gov/publications/brochurewomen/Woman_English.pdf.

Umberson, Debra, Tetyana Pudrovska, and Corinne Reczek. "Parenthood, Childlessness, and Well-Being: A Life Course Perspective." *Journal of Marriage and Family* 72 (2010): 612–29.

USDA. "Dietary Guidelines for Americans, 2020–2025." December 2020, https://www.dietaryguidelines.gov/sites/default/files/2021-03/Dietary_Guidelines_for_Americans-2020-2025.pdf.

Wade, Lisa, and Myra Marx Ferree. *Gender: Ideas, Interactions, and Institutions*. New York: W. W. Norton, 2019.

Ward, Russell A., Glenna Spitze, and Glenn Deane. "The More the Merrier? Multiple Parent–Adult Child Relations." *Journal of Marriage and Family* 71 (2009): 161–73.

Werner, Anne, and Kirsti Malterud. "Children of Parents with Alcohol Problems Performing Normality: A Qualitative Interview Study About Unmet Needs for Professional Support." *International Journal of Qualitative Studies on Health and Well-Being* 11 (2016): 1–11, 6.

Whelehan, Emelda. *Overloaded: Popular Culture and the Future of Feminism*. London, England: The Women's Press, 2000.

Whitaker, Holly. "The Patriarchy of Alcoholics Anonymous." December 27, 2019, https://www.nytimes.com/2019/12/27/opinion/alcoholics-anonymous-women.html.

White, Aaron M., I-Jen P. Castle, Ralph W. Hingson, and Patricia A. Powell. "Using Death Certificates to Explore Changes in Alcohol-Related Mortality in the United States, 1999 to 2017." *Alcoholism: Clinical and Experimental Research* 44 (2020): 178–87.

White, Aaron, I-Jen P. Castle, Chiung M. Chen, Mariela Shirley, Deidra Roach, and Ralph Hingson. "Converging Patterns of Alcohol Use and Related Outcomes